New Frontiers in Translation Studies

Series Editor

Defeng Li, Center for Studies of Translation, Interpreting and Cognition, University of Macau, Macao SAR, China

Translation Studies as a discipline has witnessed the fastest growth in the last 40 years. With translation becoming increasingly more important in today's glocalized world, some have even observed a general translational turn in humanities in recent years. The New Frontiers in Translation Studies aims to capture the newest developments in translation studies, with a focus on:

- Translation Studies research methodology, an area of growing interest amongst translation students and teachers;
- Data-based empirical translation studies, a strong point of growth for the discipline because of the scientific nature of the quantitative and/or qualitative methods adopted in the investigations; and
- Asian translation thoughts and theories, to complement the current Eurocentric translation studies.

Submission and Peer Review:

The editor welcomes book proposals from experienced scholars as well as young aspiring researchers. Please send a short description of 500 words to the editor Prof. Defeng Li at Springernfits@gmail.com and Springer Senior Publishing Editor Rebecca Zhu: Rebecca.zhu@springernature.com. All proposals will undergo peer review to permit an initial evaluation. If accepted, the final manuscript will be peer reviewed internally by the series editor as well as externally (single blind) by Springer ahead of acceptance and publication.

Raquel Lázaro Gutiérrez · Cristina Álvaro Aranda
Editors

New Trends in Healthcare Interpreting Studies

An Updated Review of Research in the Field

Springer

Editors
Raquel Lázaro Gutiérrez
FITISPos-UAH Group
University of Alcalá
Madrid, Spain

Cristina Álvaro Aranda
FITISPos-UAH Group
University of Alcalá
Madrid, Spain

ISSN 2197-8689 ISSN 2197-8697 (electronic)
New Frontiers in Translation Studies
ISBN 978-981-99-2960-3 ISBN 978-981-99-2961-0 (eBook)
https://doi.org/10.1007/978-981-99-2961-0

This Springer imprint is published by the registered company Springer Nature Singapore Pte Ltd.
The registered company address is: 152 Beach Road, #21-01/04 Gateway East, Singapore 189721, Singapore

Contents

Contributors

Carmen Acosta Vicente University of Helsinki, Helsinki, Finland

Michaela Albl-Mikasa Zurich University of Applied Sciences, Winterthur, Switzerland

Cristina Álvaro Aranda University of Alcalá, Madrid, Spain

Noelia Burdeus-Domingo Valencian International University, Valencia, Spain

Ineke H. M. Crezee Auckland University of Technology, Auckland, New Zealand

Ana Isabel Foulquié-Rubio Universidad de Murcia, Murcia, Spain

Yunduan Gao University of Auckland, Auckland, New Zealand; Gaoxinxi District, Chengdu, Sichuan, China

Laura Parrilla Gómez University Pablo de Olavide, Seville, Spain

Christiane Hohenstein Zurich University of Applied Sciences, Winterthur, Switzerland

Raquel Lázaro Gutiérrez University of Alcalá, Madrid, Spain

Harold Lesch Department Afrikaans and Dutch, Stellenbosch University, Cape Town, South Africa

Almudena Nevado Llopis Universidad San Jorge Campus Villanueva de Gállego, Villanueva de Gállego, Zaragoza, Spain

Elena Pérez Estevan University of Alicante, Alicante, Spain

Encarnación Postigo Pinazo University of Málaga, Málaga, Spain

Introduction to New Trends in Healthcare Interpreting Studies

Raquel Lázaro Gutiérrez and Cristina Álvaro Aranda

Interpreting studies have exponentially grown over the years propelled by the realities of multicultural societies which, amongst other factors, include constant waves of immigration and the subsequent allocation of newly arrived citizens in their host countries—a process entailing public service access and provision. Communicative interactions between users who do not speak the same language as public service providers have been largely studied in different settings belonging to the field PSIT (Public Service Translation and Interpreting), ranging from police, asylum, legal, educational, or, the focus of this volume, healthcare contexts.

For example, several manuals for the training or self-training of healthcare interpreters have been published, such as Abraham et al. (2004), Angelelli (2019), Bancroft (2016), Swabey (2012), or the series by Crezee et al. (2013, 2015, 2016a, b). Research on healthcare interpreting has traditionally been addressed together with translation, as in Meng (2019), Montalt (2012), Valera (2015), and the monographs which deal exclusively with healthcare interpreting date back from almost a decade ago (Pöchhacker and Schlesinger (eds.) 2005; Dörte 2009; Lázaro Gutiérrez 2012; Nicodemus 2014), with the recent exception of Souza and Fragkou (2020), whose handbook consists of a compendium of chapters about research on medical interpreting, including educational, ethical, pedagogical, and specialised aspects.

This volume stems from the wish and needs to further advance knowledge on healthcare interpreting and to reflect on new trends in the field. It contains contributions from Europe (Spain, Finland and Switzerland), Australia (New Zealand),

R. Lázaro Gutiérrez (✉) · C. Álvaro Aranda
University of Alcalá, Madrid, Spain
e-mail: raquel.lazaro@uah.es

C. Álvaro Aranda
e-mail: cristina.alvaroa@uah.es

R. Lázaro Gutiérrez and C. Álvaro Aranda (eds.), *New Trends in Healthcare Interpreting Studies*, New Frontiers in Translation Studies,
https://doi.org/10.1007/978-981-99-2961-0_1

Africa (South Africa) and North America (Canada). Although by no means exhaustive, it offers an updated insight into research and state of the art in healthcare interpreting. Aspects such as the analysis of authentic data (conversations); the increasing presence of technology in the fields of research, training and practice; the need to acquire and deploy a wide array of competences, including many that go beyond the main classical interpreting skills; the influence of and the mapping of, on the one hand, existing related literature, and, on the other, training and service provision are recurrently covered in the eight chapters of this monograph.

In the last years, scientific production in healthcare interpreting has revolved around interpreters' competences and training needs, and the description of actual practice using a variety of methodologies. In times when gathering authentic data is increasingly difficult due to bureaucratic complications and a greater awareness about research ethics, privacy, and personal data protection, recording conversations for ulterior analysis becomes more difficult. Obtaining mandatory permission nowadays usually implies presenting complex dossiers to ethics' committees and waiting for months for answers which might be negative. Angelelli (2017) explains that interpreter-mediated healthcare encounters are private in nature and patients are vulnerable. Thus, because of its characteristics, access (and recording) of these encounters is complicated. This provokes researchers to find other means of analysis that are based on other kinds of data, or resorting to reduced datasets.

One example of the latter is the study by Fovo and Eugenia (2017), who, by means of a case study, uses conversation analysis with a focus on interactional sociolinguistics to study how interpreters promote or exclude emotions. In the same vein, Merlini (2017) also analyses one interpreter-mediated conversation from three different theoretical constructs (conversational dominance, verbal politeness, and empathy) to conclude that such a combined approach improves data interpretation, offering a multiple-angled view.

Studies based on surveys and interviews are also very useful to find out about perceptions. Particularly interesting is the one developed by Van De Geuchte and Van Vaerenbergh (2017) in that they surveyed two different groups of subjects: intercultural mediators and social interpreters. Whereas in many countries there is no difference between these two kinds of professionals, in Belgium both profiles exist and are described separately. These two authors found out that, whereas mediators felt they could adopt a variety of different roles, interpreters failed to abide by their code of ethics, which might reveal their role is too narrow for the tasks they need to perform. Complemented by a survey on healthcare professionals, this study also showed that the expectations of healthcare staff about interpreters' roles and performance correspond more to the profile of intercultural mediators. Sanz Moreno (2018) also surveyed healthcare professionals in a study that combined questionnaires and interviews. Her aim was to find out about their experiences with different modalities of interpretation and to know about their opinions on the skills interpreters should possess. Other authors using questionnaires are Pokorn (2017), who investigated about the spatial positioning of healthcare interpreters in Slovenia, Hommes et al. (2018), who surveyed American Sign Language interpreters, and Ross (2020), who surveyed healthcare professionals about (non)professional interpreting in Turkey.

Burdeus Domingo (2019) developed an interview-based study in which she contrasted healthcare interpreting provisions in Montreal and Barcelona. Another study based on interviews is that of Granhagen Jungner et al. (2018), who, after surveying interpreters with experience in the paediatric oncology practice, managed to describe different strategies that they deployed to manage the bilingual conversation. Leanza et al. (2017) also analysed the views of healthcare professionals about the tasks and roles of interpreters, this time in Canada and by means of focus groups. They found out that interpreters were not considered members of the healthcare staff. Contrarily, they were portrayed as controllable instruments that serve other professionals' purposes. Álvaro Aranda (2020) used participant observation, field notes and interviews to describe the roles and tasks of healthcare interpreters. Moreno Bello (2020) also used interviews, this time to analyse the importance of the interpreter's role as a cultural broker in healthcare literacy processes in Kenya.

In the last years, research in healthcare interpreting has paid attention to specific settings. For instance, Lundin et al. (2018) carried out a descriptive study about interpreting in emergency healthcare. Perhaps one of the most important ones is that of mental health. In this area, we would like to highlight the contrastive study of Burdeus Domingo (2018), who compares service provision in Spain and Canada. In Europe, the project MHEALTH4ALL (Mental HEALTH 4 ALL: Development and implementation of a digital platform for the promotion of access to mental healthcare for low language proficient third-country nationals in Europe; https://www.mhealth4all.eu/) will be running until the end of 2024 and will explore, amongst other communication facilitators, interpreting in the domain of mental health.

Research in interpreting in general has experimented with a cognitive turn in the last decade. In this area, Albl-Mikasa (2019) analyses a corpus of 19 interpreter-mediated healthcare encounters from the prism of situated cognition and functional pragmatics. She concludes that interpreters base their decisions on a deep understanding of the healthcare professional action plan and interaction aims, which helps them towards effective performance. From a different angle, Angelelli studies, as Albl-Mikasa (2019) did, discourse coordination and interpreting-deviant roles of interpreters in recordings of authentic encounters.

From 2020 onwards, we witness the proliferation of articles focusing on remote modalities of interpreting, such as the ones by De Boe (2020, 2021), who studied simulations of medical encounters with interpreters through video links. Cotret et al. (2020), using a methodology that combined literature review, focus groups and interviews, developed a guide to the planning and practice of remote public service interpreting in Quebec. Havelka (2020) analysed video-mediated remote interpreting in Austria by means of a pilot project that combined analysis of authentic interactions and interviews. In Spain, the project PRAGMACOR (Corpus pragmatics and telephone interpreting: analysis of face-threatening acts; https://fitisposgrupo.web.uah.es/investigacion/) also focuses on remote interpreting, in particular, in three-way conversations in service provision. The corpus compiled for this project includes an important subcorpus of conversations within the healthcare domain.

Interestingly enough, several authors have given a second opportunity to their datasets and have turned their recordings, usually compiled one or two decades before in the frame of wider studies, into digital corpuses of transcriptions. A couple of examples of studies which perform corpus analysis are those by Angelelli (2017) and Pöllabauer (2017). Castagnoli and Niemants (2018) also use corpus analysis to contrast on-site and remote interpreting, breaking the ground for a very promising research area, and Falbo (2018) presents the compilation and characteristics of two different corpora, CorIT (Italian Television Interpreting Corpus) and CorILex (Legal Interpreting Corpus), with the aim of exploring the role of interpreting corpora within corpus linguistics. Niemants (2018) processes the corpus AIM with the software EXMARaLDA and ELAN to extract lexical patterns and align audio and transcriptions. Regarding sign language, Major and McKee (2020) carried out a terminological study in which they analysed a corpus of deaf New Zealand Sign Language users' accounts of women's health-related experiences. Their aim was to examine the language forms they used to communicate such topics to identify vocabulary to be included in interpreter training.

Sánchez Ramos (2017) also uses corpus analysis, but this time to train interpreters and develop their documentation skills. Also related to technology are the different training proposals that focus on remote interpreting modalities (over the phone and through video links). Some of these are those by Albl-Mikasa and Eingrieber (2018) and the project SHIFT in Orality (Amato et al. 2018). Very revolutionary is the proposal by Eser et al. (2020), who describes a learning experience based on the use of three-dimensional virtual reality glasses to train healthcare interpreters in immersive simulated environments.

Regarding the teaching and learning of healthcare interpreting, it is worth mentioning the works by Niemants and Stokoe (2017) and Dal Fovo and Eugenia (2018), who apply the CARM (Conversation Analytic Role-play Method) to train healthcare interpreters. This method involves the use of authentic data and its analysis by means of conversation analysis. Authenticity is also brought to the healthcare interpreting classroom in pedagogical experiments based on situated learning (Sanz Moreno 2017), or the interprofessional education (IPE) strategy (Hlavac and Harrison 2021).

Thematically, the contributions of this volume touch upon several relevant topics echoing current research interests in healthcare interpreting previously described, and also bring to the fore new lenses to approach them. These include distinguishing features, education and training, the status of healthcare interpreting in particular national contexts, demographics, new technologies, and specialised contexts in health delivery.

Albl-Mikasa and Hohenstein open the volume with an analysis of healthcare interpreting from a discourse analysis framework that incorporates both cognitive and social dimensions, as found in the Heidelberg School of Interpreting Studies, which is conveniently updated with insights into Functional Pragmatics. The authors defend that a healthcare interpreter's domain-specific, discourse-related and institutional knowledge affects the course of an interaction, even impeding its intended purposes at higher and lower levels. To illustrate this, Albl-Mikasa and Hohenstein closely examine two extracts from a corpus of video-recorded authentic provider-patient-encounters with the intervention of an interpreter that occurred in a hospital.

They convene that healthcare interpreters must understand institutional knowledge and related language (e.g., expressions and lexical constructions) in order to help providers to complete their goals and action plans.

The education section is inaugurated by Noelia Burdeus-Domingo. She presents a didactic proposal for teaching cultural competence in healthcare interpreting training programmes drawing on the Purnell model, which finds its origin in the medical and nursing education spheres and is further complemented by the author's recommendations to suit the reality of healthcare interpreting practices. More precisely, Burdeus Domingo proposes several collaborative activities divided into 12 sections that allow interpreter trainers and learners to reflect on cross-cultural communication issues between local and target communities. These include, but are not limited to, family roles and organisations, death rituals and spirituality, and health practices. By aligning healthcare interpreting training with a framework used to train other healthcare profiles, Burdeus-Domingo sets the ground for future interprofessional collaboration in triad encounters.

Postigo Pinazo and Parrilla Gómez also reflect on healthcare interpreter training, but this time considering the unstoppable advent of new technologies in professional interpreting practice and university education. More particularly, the authors assess the potential of Otter.ai and Amberscript, two audio transcriptions (i.e., speech-to-text) tools. To evaluate their features, Postigo Pinazo and Parrilla Gómez use a corpus of real conversations obtained in a hospital setting, which are analysed using both programmes and subsequently compared with a manual transcription performed by the authors. Although background noise, long sentences and interruptions negatively affect software performance, both tools capture the most significant information in short recordings, including terminology, procedures and dates.

For their part, Nevado Llopis and Foulquié Rubio describe the state of healthcare interpreting the training in Spanish universities to establish if existing programmes cater to its peculiarities. They perform an online search to pinpoint the Spanish universities offering T&I, which is complemented by focus groups involving interpreters, lecturers, and heads of departments and directors of T&I degrees. Some problematic areas inferred from this research include a generalised lack of psychological training on how to face challenging situations and the provision of minority languages in the curricula. The authors advocate for mixed methodologies in healthcare interpreting training, which ideally would bring students closer to the actual healthcare interpreting practice and involve trainees and/or professionals from the health community, amongst other aspects. To help interpret students and trainers, they introduce a virtual platform derived from the REACTMe project (Research & Action and Training in Medical Interpreting), which includes relevant training materials.

Similarly, Crezee and Gao provide an overview of healthcare interpreting as a professional activity and educational field in New Zealand, one of the first countries offering non-language specific courses for healthcare interpreters at the tertiary level. The contribution first examines some studies approaching training programmes in the country, with particular emphasis on situated learning, self-reflection and peer feedback activities, shared interprofessional learning and idiomatic language. Subsequently, and drawing on a dataset of participant observations of interpreter-mediated interactions and interviews with stakeholders used in Gao's doctoral thesis, the authors observe what happens in real interactions with trained interpreters in the healthcare setting. They describe a set of demands placed on interpreters and the various controls they employ before and during assignments to respond to such demands (e.g., explaining the health system). This allows inferring useful implications for interpreting education programmes, such as including (semi-)authentic materials, field observations and role-plays involving health providers.

Adopting a diachronic perspective, Lesch evaluates the situation of healthcare interpreting in public hospitals in the Western Cape, South Africa. This geographical context is not only influenced by the influx of migrants from other countries, but also by the coexistence of different official languages, and the subsequent multilingual language policy in place, which resorts to translation and interpreting services for support. Against this backdrop, Lesch assesses the progress of healthcare interpreting from different angles, including ad hoc practices, telephone and on-site interpreting, interpreting in mental health, and role shifting (i.e., demands placed on healthcare interpreters and affecting their role, such as acting as lay counsellors). Although some limited inroads have been made in the field, the author indicates that further improvements are still essential to guarantee the implementation of efficient interpreting healthcare services that give non-English speaking patients a voice.

Moving away from education and training, Pérez Estevan explores the understudied area of healthcare interpreting in end-of-life encounters in Spain, with a special emphasis on the psychotherapists' views on the tasks and role of interpreters working in the field. To do so, Pérez Estevan combines surveys and in-depth interviews that yield interesting results. Amongst these, it must be noted that, rather than linguistic duties, providers underline the importance of tasks related to emotions and the doctor-patient relationship, including confidentiality, trust, and respect for other's feelings. Additionally, briefing and debriefing sessions are identified as key areas deserving further attention. While briefing fosters understanding of the interpreter's role and helps to structure the delivery of bad news or difficult information, debriefing allows interpreters to vent their emotions and safeguard their psychological well-being, which is particularly relevant after a patient's death.

Demographics are another key element explored in the volume. In this sense, Acosta Vicente approaches the issue of *gender* in healthcare interpreting. Drawing on a sample of relevant journals and monographs in interpreting studies and adjacent disciplines, she explores how the literature problematises gender-related issues and identifies four key areas: i. role differences based on the interpreter's gender, ii. gendered behaviours and outside perceptions of interpreters, iii. interpreter's management of gendered language or discourse, and iv. gender dynamics between participants in interpreter-mediated interactions. Acosta Vicente calls for greater attention from researchers into the implications of gender, as it could improve the delivery of quality interpreting services (e.g., the interpreter's gender may impact the patient's level of comfort to disclose personal information).

As it can be deduced from our preliminary words, this edited volume aims to advance knowledge on healthcare interpreting and reflect on new research trends.

This interesting collection of papers will greatly benefit scholars, students, and practitioners in the field of healthcare interpreting by providing an updated revision of different research trends in just one volume, thus helping us to establish where we are and where we are headed to.

References

Abraham, Diana, Nelson Cabral, and Anita Tancredi, eds. 2004. *A Handbook for Trainers: Language Interpreting in the Healthcare Sector*. Toronto: Healthcare Interpretation Network.

Albl-Mikasa, Michaela, and Monika Eingrieber. 2018. Training video interpreters for refugee languages in the German-speaking DACH countries. *Fitispos International Journal* 5: 33–44.

Albl-Mikasa, Michaela. 2019. Acting upon background of understanding rather than role. Shifting the focus from the interactional to the inferential dimension of (medical) dialogue interpreting. *Translation: Cognition & Behavior* 2(2): 241–262.

Álvaro Aranda, Cristina. 2020. Analysing the healthcare interpreter's role in the "in-between". An exploratory study of patient-interpreter spoken interactions in a hospital setting. *SKASE (Journal of Translation and Interpretation)* 13 (2): 22–37.

Amato, Amalia; Nicoletta Spinolo & María Jesús González Rodríguez (eds.) 2018. Handbook of remote interpreting—SHIFT in Orality. Bologna: Universitá de Bologna

Andres, Dörte., and Sonja Pöllabauer, eds. 2009. *Spürst Du, wie der Bauch rauf-runter? Fachdolmetschen im Gesundheitsbereich. Is everything all topsy turvy in your tummy? Healthcare Interpreting*. München: Meidenbauer.

Angelelli, Claudia V. 2017. Can ethnographic findings become corpus-studies data? A researcher's ethical, practical and scientific dilemmas. *The Interpreters' Newsletter* 22: 1–15.

Angelelli, Claudia V. 2019. *Healthcare interpreting explained*. London: Routledge.

Angelelli, Claudia V. 2020. Who is talking now? role expectations and role materializations in interpreter-mediated healthcare encounters. *Communication & Medicine* 15 (2): 123–134.

Bancroft, Marjory A., Sofia Garcia Beyaert; Katharine Allen. 2016. Giovanna Carriero-Contreras & Denis Socarras-Estrada. *The Medical Interpreter. A Foundation Textbook for Medical Interpreting*. Columbia: Culture & Language Press.

Burdeus-Domingo, Noelia. 2018. Interpreting in mental health. An effective communication facilitation practice. *Current Trends in Translation Teaching and Learning E—CTTL E* 5: 71–105.

Burdeus-Domingo, Noelia. 2019. Structuring public service interpreting. The interpreters bank model as an organised response to communication needs. *Fitispos International Journal* 6: 46–61.

Castagnoli, Sara & Natacha Niemants. 2018). Corpora worth creating: A pilot study on telephone interpreting inTRAlinea Special Issue: Bendazzoli, Claudio; Mariachiara Russo & Bart Defrancq (eds.) 'New Findings in Corpus-based Interpreting Studies.'

Cotret, François René, de Andrée-Anne Beaudoin-Julien, and Yvan Leanza. 2020. Implementing and managing remote public service interpreting in response to COVID-19 and other challenges of globalization. *Meta* 65 (3): 618–642.

Crezee, Ineke. 2013. *Introduction to Healthcare for Interpreters and Translators*. Amsterdam: John Benjamins.

Crezee, Ineke, Holly Mikkelson, and Laura Monzon-Storey. 2015. *Introduction to Healthcare for Spanish-speaking Interpreters and Translators*. Amsterdam: John Benjamins.

Crezee, Ineke, Nawar Gailani, and Anna N. Gailani. 2016a. *Introduction to Healthcare for Arabic-sepaking Interpreters and Translators*. Amsterdam: John Benjamins.

Crezee, Ineke, and Eva N. S. Ng. 2016b. *Introduction to Healthcare for Chinese-speaking Interpreters and Translators*. Amsterdam: John Benjamins

Dal Fovo, Eugenia. 2017. Good health across languages: How access to healthcare by non-Italian speaking patients is ensured in Italy. A case study. *Lingue Culture Mediazioni/Languages Cultures Mediation* 4 (1): 33–55.
De Boe, Esther. 2020. Remote interpreting in dialogic settings. A methodological framework for investigating the impact of telephone and video interpreting on quality in healthcare interpreting. In: Saalets, Heidi & Gert Brône (eds.) Linking up with video. *Perspectives on Interpreting Practice And Research.* Amsterdam: John Benjamins: 77–105.
De Boe, Esther. 2021. Management of overlapping speech in remote healthcare interpreting. *The Interpreters' Newsletter* 26: 139-157
De Geuchte, Van, Sofie, and Vaerenbergh Leona. 2017. Interpreting in Flemish Hospitals: Interpreters' View and Healthcare Workers' Expectations. *CLINA* 3 (1): 117–144.
Eser, Oktay, Miranda Lai, and Fatih Saltan. 2020. The affordances and challenges of wearable technologies for training public service interpreters. *Interpreting (International Journal of Research and Practice in Interpreting)* 22 (2): 288–308.
Falbo, Caterina. 2018. La collecte de corpus d'interprétation: Un défi permanent. *Meta* 63: 649–664.
Fovo, Dal, and Eugenia. 2018. The use of dialogue interpreting corpora in healthcare interpreter training: Taking stock. *The Interpreters' Newsletter* 23: 83–113.
Havelka, Ivana. 2020. Video-mediated remote interpreting in healthcare. Analysis of an Austrian pilot project. *Babel* 66 (2): 326–345.
Hlavac, Jim & Claire Harrison. 2021. Interpreter-mediated doctor-patient interactions. Interprofessional education in the training of future interpreters and doctors. *Perspectives: Studies in Translation Theory and Practice* 29 (4): 572–590.
Hommes, Rachel E., Amy I. Borash, Kari A. Hartwig and Donna DeGracia. 2018 American sign language interpreters perceptions of barriers to healthcare communication in deaf and hard of hearing. *Journal of Community Health* 43 (5): 956-961.
Ji, Meng, Mustapha Taibi, and Ineke Crezee, eds. 2019. *Multicultural Health Translation, Interpreting and Communication.* London: Routledge.
Jungner, Granhagen, Johanna, Elisabet Tiselius, Klas Blomgren, Kim Lützén, and Pernilla Pergert. 2018. The interpreter's voice. Carrying the bilingual conversation in interpreter-mediated consultations in pediatric oncology care. *Patient Education and Counselling* 102 (4): 656–662.
Lázaro Gutiérrez, Raquel. 2012. *La interpretación en el ámbito sanitario: Estudio de la asimetría en consultas médicas.* Saarbrücken: Editorial Académica Española, LAP LAMBERT Academic Publishing.
Leanza, Yvan, Rizkallah, Elias, Michaud-Labonté, Thomas and Brisset, Camille. 2017. From concern for patients to a quest for information. How medical socialization shapes family physicians' representations of interpreters. *Interpreting (International Journal of Research and Practice in Interpreting)* 19(2): 232–259.
Lundin, Christina, Emina Hadziabdic and Katarina Hjelm. 2018. Language interpretation conditions and boundaries in multilingual and multicultural emergency healthcare. *BMC International Health and Human Rights* 18: 1.
Major, George, and Rachel McKee. 2020. Deaf women's health vocabulary, challenges for interpreters working in a language of limited diffusion. *International Journal of Interpreter Education (IJIE)* 12 (2): 1–18.
Merlini, Raffaela. 2017. Interactional data through the kaleidoscope of analytical perspectives: Reassembling the picture. *Dragoman* 5 (7): 17–31.
Montalt i Resurrecció, Vicent and Mark Shuttleworth (eds.). 2012. Research in translation and knowledge mediation in medical and healthcare settings. Linguistica Antverpiensia, New Series (LANS) 11.
Moreno Bello, Yolanda. 2020. The interpreter as intercultural mediator in the acquisition of health literacy. A case study from Kenya. *Translation Matters* 2 (1): 70–83.
Nicodemus, Brenda, and Melanie Metzger (eds.). 2014. *Investigations in Healthcare Interpreting.* Washington DC: Gallaudet University.

Niemants, Natacha. 2018. Des enregistrements aux corpus: Transcription et extraction de données d'interprétation en milieu médical. *Meta* 63 (3): 665–694.
Niemants, Natascha, and Stokoe Elizabeth. 2017. Using the conversation analytic role-play method in healthcare interpreter education. In: Cirillo, Letizia and Natacha Niemants (eds.) *Teaching Dialogue Interpreting. Research-based proposals for higher education.* Amsterdam: John Benjamins: 294–321.
Pöchhacker, Franz & Miriam Shlesinger (eds.). 2005. Healthcare Interpreting. Discourse and Interaction. *Interpreting (International Journal of Research and Practice in Interpreting)* 7:2.
Pokorn, Nike K. 2017. There is always some spatial limitation. Spatial positioning and seating arrangement in healthcare interpreting. *TIS (Translation and Interpreting Studies)* 12 (3): 383–404.
Pöllabauer, Sonja. 2017. Issues of terminology in public service interpreting: From affordability through psychotherapy to waiting lists. In: Antonini, Rachele, Letizia Cirillo, Linda Rossato, and Ira Torresi (eds.) Non-professional Interpreting and Translation. *State of the Art and Future of an Emerging Field of Research.* Amsterdam: John Benjamins: 131–155.
Ross, Jonathan Maurice. 2020. Chinese whispers in Turkish hospitals. Doctors' views of non-professional interpreting in Eastern Turkey. *Parallèles* 32 (2): 63–81.
Salinas, Varela, María-José, and Bernd Meyer. (eds.). 2015. *Translating and Interpreting Healthcare Discourses/Traducir e interpretar en el ámbito sanitario.* Berlin: Frank & Timme.
Sánchez Ramos, María del Mar. 2017. Interpretación sanitaria y herramientas informáticas de traducción: los sistemas de gestión de corpus. Panace@ 18(46): 133–141.
Sanz Moreno, Raquel. 2017. Dilemas éticos en interpretación sanitaria. El médico entra en el aula. Panace@ 18 (46): 114–122.
Sanz Moreno, Raquel. 2018. La percepción del personal sanitario sobre la interpretación en hospitales. Estudio de caso. Panace@ 19(47): 67–75.
Souza, Isabel E. T. de V., and Effrossyni Fragkou (eds.). 2020. Handbook of research on medical interpreting. Hershey (Pennsylvania): IGI Global.
Swabey, Laurie, and Karen Malcolm. (eds.). 2012. *In Our Hands: Educating Healthcare Interpreters.* Washington DC: Gallaudet University.

Raquel Lázaro Gutiérrez is an Associate Professor in the Department of Modern Philology at the University of Alcalá and teaches the Degree in Modern Languages and Translation and the Master's Degree in Intercultural Communication and Public Service Interpreting and Translation. She has been a member of the FITISPos-UAH Research Group since 2001 and Vice-President of the European Association ENPSIT. She has been the PI of several projects such as "Corpus pragmatics and telephone interpreting", funded by the Spanish Government (2023–2026). She has participated in European research projects such as SOS-VICS (2011–2014), AHEH-Knowledge Alliances (2018–2021), or MHEALTH4ALL (2022–2025).

Cristina Álvaro Aranda is a PhD Assistant Professor at the University of Alcalá, where she teaches several subjects in the Modern Languages and Translation degree and collaborates with the Master's Degree in Intercultural Communication and Public Service Interpreting and Translation. She holds a PhD in Modern Languages and Translation focusing on healthcare interpreting from the University of Alcalá, with the distinctions of Doctor Cum Laude and International Doctorate. She is currently participating in the European research project MHEALTH4ALL. She has been a Visiting Student at Heriot-Watt University (2018) and King's College London (2019) and is a member of AFIPTISP and the FITISPos-UAH Research Group.

Community Interpreting as a Socially *and* Cognitively Situated Activity: Speech Action Patterns and Underlying Knowledge Structures in Interpreter-Mediated Medical Interactions

Michaela Albl-Mikasa and Christiane Hohenstein

1 Introduction

This paper, which addresses cognitive aspects of community interpreting (CI), was originally intended for publication in the volume featuring selected papers from the Critical Link 8 Conference which took place in Edinburgh in 2016. The volume did not materialize and, in the meantime, the introduction of the cognitive dimension into community interpreting has caught on. Having been largely ignored in community interpreting research until then (see Englund Dimitrova and Tiselius 2016; Albl-Mikasa 2019), it has since been the subject of a special thematic section of a 2019 Translation, Cognition and Behaviour issue (Tiselius and Albl-Mikasa 2019). However, it has not yet been taken up to an extent that reflects its importance. This can be gleaned from the forthcoming Routledge Handbook on Public Service Interpreting. Of the 25 chapters, only one deals with cognitive processing in community interpreting or, more precisely, monitoring, namely that of Englund Dimitrova and Tiselius. Other than that, there is no mention of the fundamental cognitive basis of CI, including inferencing, recourse to knowledge structures, cognitive processes, etc. Knowledge is only mentioned in a very general sense, i.e. referring to knowledge and skills, bridging the knowledge gap between doctors and patients, or medical and/or terminological knowledge. With this in mind, this updated version of the original paper addresses a lingering gap. It is a continuation of an introductory paper (Albl-Mikasa and Hohenstein 2017), which applied Functional Pragmatics to

M. Albl-Mikasa (✉) · C. Hohenstein
Zurich University of Applied Sciences, Winterthur, Switzerland
e-mail: michaela.albl-mikasa@zhaw.ch

R. Lázaro Gutiérrez and C. Álvaro Aranda (eds.), *New Trends in Healthcare Interpreting Studies*, New Frontiers in Translation Studies,
https://doi.org/10.1007/978-981-99-2961-0_2

medical interpreting, drawing attention to how a lack of understanding of a given institutional set-up—in terms of institutional processes and associated speech routines, linguistic procedures as well as set phrases and expressions—deprives the interpreter of common ground with the doctor (and sometimes even the patient), which is the very foundation of effective and efficient interpreting.

After providing the background for the apparent non-appraisal of the cognitive dimension and introducing a situated cognition and Functional Pragmatics perspective, which serves to highlight the significance of the interpreter's institutional, domain-specific and discourse-related knowledge, this paper presents a detailed analysis of two examples from the Swiss Basel University Hospital/Zurich University of Applied Sciences corpus of 19 video-recorded authentic doctor-patient encounters. The analysis clearly demonstrates the role knowledge plays in interpreter-mediated doctor-patient conversations (IDPC) at a higher (e.g. schemata about institutional processes) and lower (linguistic micro-structures) level. More specifically, it illustrates how the non-rendition of certain speech actions and institutional action patterns (example 1) and of seemingly trivial routine (matrix) constructions (example 2) during interpreting may affect the course of the conversation and impede its goals and purposes. The former example is a more detailed elaboration of the 2017 analysis, the latter is newly added in order to demonstrate that knowledge is key at both the macro and micro level.

2 From Social to Socio-Cognitive Interaction

It is generally accepted that interpreting is an act of pragmatic cognitive discourse processing that depends heavily on various types of linguistic and non-linguistic knowledge. Applied to community interpreting, it can be shown that medical interpreting goes way beyond coordinating turns and conveying conversational snippets, and that interpreters, in fact, enact institutional processes, if they share relevant knowledge structures.

2.1 Community Interpreting as Social Interaction

Research into what is generally referred to as "community interpreting" (Bancroft 2015: 219) and subsumes medical interpreting has predominantly focused on the descriptive analysis of discourse in interaction (DI). In fact, according to Pöchhacker, two different paradigms have evolved, the "DI paradigm" for community and the cognitive processes or "CP paradigm" for conference interpreting (Pöchhacker 2015: 66, 68). Accordingly, the focus has been on communicative interactions, conversational management and role behaviour for community interpreting and on mental processing, capacity management and strategic behaviour for conference interpreting (Albl-Mikasa 2020: 93). This separation can be traced back to the influential work of Wadensjö (1998), who placed emphasis on dialogue interpreters' coordinating (rather than simply translating) talk in social interaction. The wide-ranging consequences of this focus culminated in researchers exclusively addressing the social and interactive processes in community interpreting at the expense of the cognitive ones.

While directing the focus to socio-interactive aspects may be plausible in view of the dialogic nature of conversational proximity in community interpreting encounters, the utter exclusion of the cognitive dimension is less so. In fact, there are some inconsistencies in the theoretical foundation. Wadensjö (2001) established the approach by adopting discourse analysis as a framework and making particular reference to Schiffrin. Accordingly, discourse analysis, "a vast and somewhat vague subfield" (Schiffrin 1994: viii), assumes some underlying model of communication, be it (a) a code model, (b) an inferential model or (c) an interactional model of communication. Wadensjö explains that her own assumed model of communication is an interactional one and that her focus is therefore on the "interpreter-mediated encounter, and not interpreting (as, say, an individual's transmission of the thoughts of others) or the interpreter (as, say, the individual as displayer of the intentions of others)" (2001: 189). As such, she excludes interpreters and their intentions or, in cognitive terms, the inferential side of interpreting. This in itself is incontestable, in that a discourse-based approach need not necessarily be a cognitive one, because discourse analysis "has come to be used [...] to describe activities at the intersection of disciplines as diverse as sociolinguistics, psycholinguistics, philosophical linguistics and computational linguistics" (Brown and Yule 1983: viii). What is debatable, however, is that Wadensjö (2001: 187) also bases her work on and explicitly refers to van Dijk (1985), whose work is a crucial part of the cognitive foundation of interpreting and, thus, the CP paradigm.

Van Dijk and Kintsch's seminal book (1983), in particular, explains discourse comprehension in terms of strategically situated cognitive activity. It serves as the very basis for Kohn and Kalina's (1996) and Kalina's (1998) no less influential cognitive-strategic approach to interpreting, which views interpreting as strategic (bilingual) text comprehension and production processes. As such, interpreting—and translation for that matter—is not only an act of communication and textual operation, but indisputably the result of cognitive processing carried out by interpreters (and translators respectively) (Hurtado Albir and Alves 2009: 54). This insight, which spurred the cognitive turn in translation studies in the context of translation process research, is as true for community interpreting as it is for conference interpreting and was recognized in conference interpreting studies long before it was taken on board by translation studies. It implies that any type of interpreting task involves mental processes, cognitive resources, language control and capacity management as well as a variety of executive functions including verbal working memory and (divided) attention (Hervais-Adelman et al. 2015). It would, therefore, be reductionist to focus merely on the interactive dimension of the situated activity. And indeed, the general focus on interactional sociolinguistics has led to a situation where the "body of research on community interpreting has to date focused mainly on aspects of the interpreter's role in the interaction between interlocutors/participants and in the communication process" (Englund Dimitrova and Tiselius 2016: 195). To widen the scope, community interpreting is better described not just as a "socially situated activity" (Pöchhacker 2015: 68), but as a socially situated *cognitive* activity, which clearly includes the cognitive processing dimension. The aim of this paper is to analyze medical interpreting within a discourse analysis framework that is both cognitive and social. Such a framework can be found in the "cognitive and pragmatic discourse model of interpreting", which has become the cornerstone of what Pöchhacker called the "Heidelberg School" (2012: 19) of Interpreting Studies.

2.2 Community Interpreting as Situated Cognitive Activity

The Heidelberg School's cognitive and pragmatic discourse model of interpreting is based on a large body of evidence from psycholinguistics and cognitive psychology (as compiled by Kintsch and van Dijk 1983 and others). Applied, in particular, by Kohn and Kalina (1996), Kalina (1998), Braun (2004) and Albl-Mikasa (2007), it centres around the view that interpreters' understanding of a source text is achieved by creating a 'mental model' during their pragmatic engagement in a meaning negotiating 'discourse' event. This involves "strategic processes of continuous and cyclic utterance meaning formation (including monitoring and revision) based on linguistic as well as world-related knowledge" (Braun and Kohn 2012: 190).

From this perspective, the core assumption is that (medical) interpreters (as well as all other participants in the encounter) are guided not just by the bottom-up speech signals they receive, but just as much by knowledge, expectations and inferences activated top-down. Interpreters' performance is greatly determined by the mental representation or model they can construct when processing an encounter, which, in turn, depends on their linguistic, domain-based and discourse-specific knowledge and the extent to which they are able to integrate it from their long-term memory into the mental representation unfolding in their working memory. Concurrently, the processing is heavily influenced by expectations generated in the process as well as by factors from the situational context.

As is known from social constructivist analyses of foreign language use and learning, cognitive processes are also determined by the individual's own developmental learning history and performance requirements, which affect attitude, motivation, self-image and goals (Kohn 2011: 72, 74, 80). This puts into perspective the emphasis which has been placed, within the DI paradigm, on interpreters' agency and profound effect upon communication dynamics (e.g. Angelelli 2004; Wadensjö 1998). As Ozolins (2015: 327) points out, this focus was put forward as a criticism of the long-cherished concepts of impartiality, neutrality and invisibility that form part of the conduit model of interpreting. From a cognitive perspective, however, community interpreters may or may not see themselves as neutral players, they may or may not strive for invisibility and they may act more actively or more passively, depending on a great many influencing factors as mentioned above (Albl-Mikasa 2020). A major factor lies in the availability of background knowledge, which is

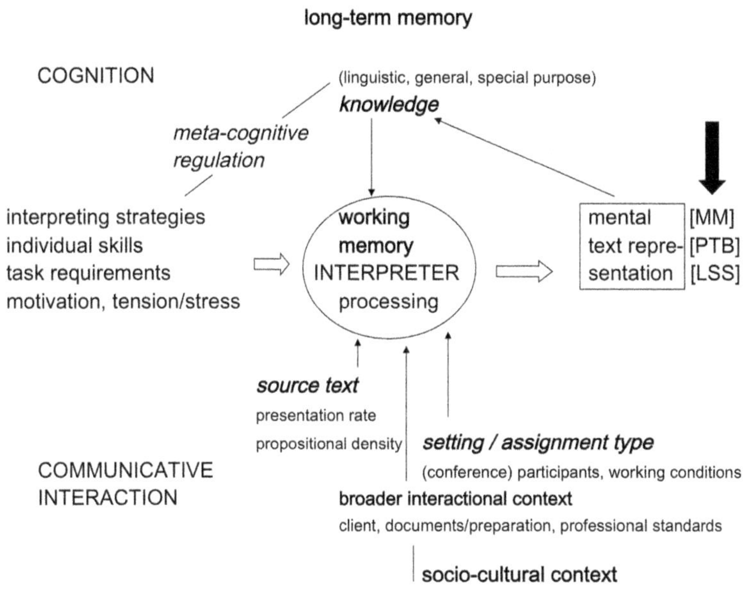

Fig. 1 Interpreting (comprehension process) as situated cognition (Albl-Mikasa 2014: 73)

required for interpreters to act upon their requirements and goals. Situational factors may also prove restrictive. In mental healthcare settings, for instance, it is much more difficult for interpreters to remain uninvolved, even if they personally strive to assume a conduit-like role in the encounter (Bot 2003). The following model (see Fig. 1) summarizes the Heidelberg School approach by depicting coherence building in the interpreting process. This encompasses the bottom-up and top-down interdependence of mental and situational inputs, along with related inferential processes, involving the construction of a mental representation of the processed input on three different levels (LSS: language surface structures; PTB: propositional textbase; MM: mental model).

An application to dialogue interpreting is illustrated in the following graph (Fig. 2):

This model illustrates how interpreters' background knowledge exerts top-down influence on their performance, how experience is gained during the interpreting performance and feeds back into knowledge and competence building, and how this overall process is influenced bottom-up by situational factors. These factors, in turn, reside on three different levels: the immediate conversational situation, the institutional setting and the general regional and cultural background (for details see Albl-Mikasa 2020). Most importantly, the model highlights how knowledge structures as part of a person's competence determine communication and, with it, the interpreter's performance and how this applies to all parties to the conversation, as each interlocutor's performance depends on available or accessible knowledge structures.

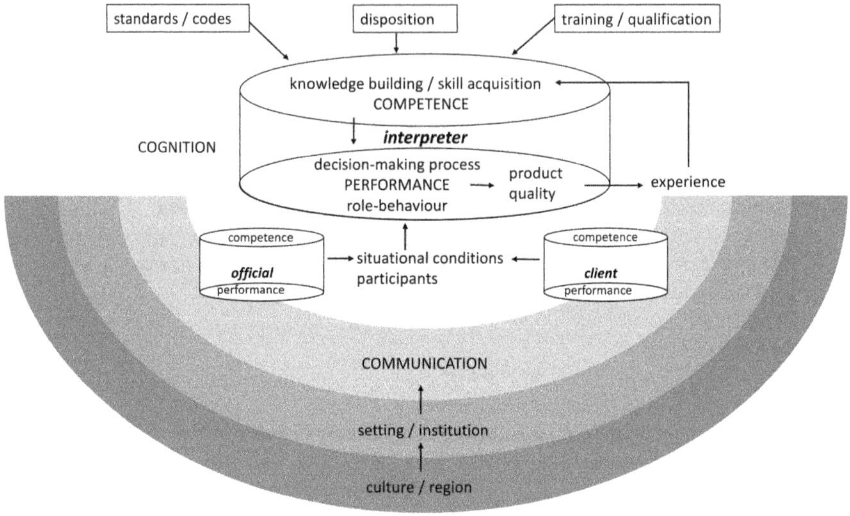

Fig. 2 Dialogue interpreting as a situated cognitive activity (Albl-Mikasa 2020: 96)

In order to account for the pragmatic dimension of the Heidelberg School's cognitive and pragmatic discourse model of interpreting, Functional Pragmatics (FP) can be integrated into the theoretical framework (Albl-Mikasa 2019), because "discourse analysis within this framework of functional pragmatics" includes "the actor's mental activities and their knowledge" (Bührig 2005: 149). FP conceives of language as a form-function nexus that is anchored in reality as societal practice and allows for a knowledge-based appropriation of reality (Redder 2008: 133, 135). Each language has its own linguistic procedures reflecting societal and institutional practices appropriating reality in specific ways. In this view, the use of language is tantamount to the processing of socially evolved action patterns and related knowledge structures. In other words, FP considers language to be linguistic action that is based on knowledge about socially and institutionally evolved action patterns. Application of knowledge is then not simply a matter of linguistic externalization or of knowledge-sharing, but is discursive action, both linguistic and non-linguistic (Meyer 2004: 46). In more tangible terms, health professionals bring to an encounter an action plan comprised of verbal and non-verbal action patterns, which are verbalized in keeping with the overall purpose of an encounter and in line with the general institutional structure and societal goal (Bührig 2005: 147). Against this backdrop of a purposeful interplay of verbal and non-verbal action patterns, an FP component makes it possible to explain the advantages community interpreters can reap when "pattern knowledge" (Redder 2008: 138) is available to act as a basis for top-down inferencing and anticipation as well as bottom-up coherence building and comprehension. At the same time, it points to potential adverse effects on communication when such knowledge is part of the competence of only one party to the dialogue or encounter. In the model in Fig. 2, the FP dimension is an integral part of the interlocutors' competence.

3 Knowledge Structures in (Interpreted) Doctor-Patient Communication

In interpreted doctor-patient communication (IDPC), the course of interaction is determined by the cognitive processing of all three parties and the respective knowledge they bring to bear on the situation as illustrated in Fig. 2. It is generally assumed that the participants are in an asymmetrical knowledge constellation. Especially the unequal distribution of knowledge between doctor and patient has often been described as resulting in a communicative relationship between an "expert" and a "lay person", when, in fact, it is more accurate to speak of the patient not as a "lay person", but as a "non-expert" within an institution (Hartog 1994, 2006: 176f, Redder 2008: 150). This is because patients, in their capacity as a client seeking counsel from the institution, carry both general and more specific first-hand empirical knowledge of institutional structures and processes, termed 'first-order knowledge'. Doctors, as agents of the institution, carry both 'first-order' and systematically acquired 'second-order' expert and institutional knowledge (Ehlich and Rehbein 1977, 1986; Redder 2008: 145–146, 150). Second-order knowledge (or "institutional knowledge Level 2", Bührig 2009: 152) includes insights into institutional structures, decision-making processes and action patterns for specific institutional purposes, with which clients/patients are not usually familiar. The more frequently patients are involved in medical encounters in hospitals and with doctors, experiencing testing and treatment processes, the better their understanding of related procedures and terminology becomes. Patients may either acquire 'semi-professional' knowledge during the course of an illness and, thus, some elements of 'second-order' expert knowledge, or 'pseudo-professional' knowledge, i.e. 'first-order' knowledge in the guise of 'second-order' knowledge, which is reflected in patients' usage of medical expressions, but does not come with an understanding of the underlying medical notions or explanatory background (Löning 1994).

Interpreters, by contrast, lack second-order knowledge in medical encounters: They may not be too familiar with the institutional processes or areas of responsibility defined within the hospital in which their interpreting assignment takes place. Nor may they be highly knowledgeable regarding the procedures in place or medical subject matter and terminology involved in the specific case. This may, in fact, be a reason why plurilingual family members and ad hoc in-house staff interpreters are sometimes better equipped for the interpreting task. Family members may have substantial knowledge relevant to the case on the basis of their close relationship with the patient and frequent visits to the hospital or talks with the doctors concerned (Rosenberg et al. 2008), i.e. first-order knowledge in part overlapping with the patient's. Similarly, in-house medical staff members' "institutional and technical knowledge can be an asset for their interpreting activities" (Martínez-Gómez 2015: 422), i.e. they share second-order institutional knowledge to some extent and have first-order knowledge from their experience.

3.1 *Types of Interaction in Doctor-Patient Communication (DPC)*

Knowledge is, thus, a term covering a wide range of matters, be it knowledge of the medical subject and terminology, of the wider institution and its processes, or of specific DPC action patterns and discourse structures. The former is dealt with by Creeze (2013), for instance, who emphasizes the need for an understanding of and background in healthcare rather than mere terminological knowledge. The latter is the subject of this paper. We will concentrate on the actual IDPC encounter and on knowledge of its specific set-up and how this is reflected in speech. To start with, each encounter is embedded into a specific purposeful process and is structured accordingly. Doctor-patient communication differentiates principally between 'initial medical interviews' and 'follow-up encounters' (see Fig. 3), depending on whether or not the doctor and patient have had previous interactions, i.e. whether or not a joint 'pre-history' of former medical encounters has been established.

First encounters or *initial medical interviews* take place when a general practitioner or medical specialist has yet to identify the illness a patient suffers from. This type of doctor-patient communication is often dubbed an 'anamnestic medical interview' due to its focus on reconstructing the patient's medical history, even though physical examination, diagnosis and counselling may take place within the same encounter. A substantial part of the encounter will revolve around establishing the patient's medical history, including family members' serious illnesses up to the point where her/his current ailments started. The internal structure of this conversational type is characterized by specific question types on the part of the doctor and narrative stretches on the part of the patient. If a serious illness is suspected or has been diagnosed and the patient is referred to a medical specialist, the specialist will once again seek to compile the personal medical history, restarting the anamnesis (see Bührig and Meyer 2009: 191).

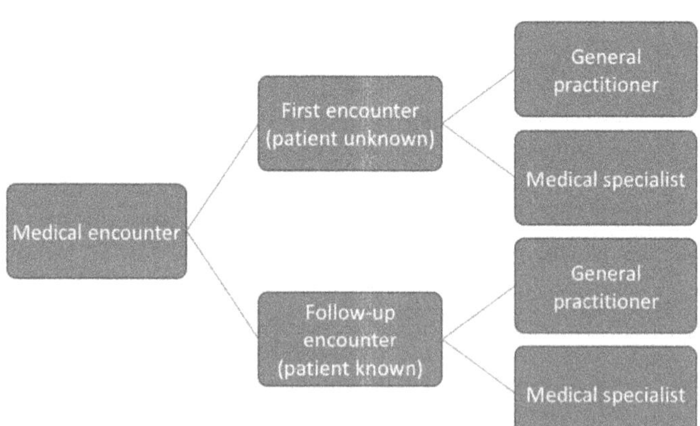

Fig. 3 Basic types of doctor-patient interaction (see Rehbein and Löning 1995)

The second discourse type, the *follow-up encounter*, includes all types of doctor-patient communication where patients are in the process of being treated or checked up on against the backdrop of a known medical history and illness. In these cases, the patient is known to the doctor, and medical records carrying information on the diagnoses, subsequent treatments and their successes are available. Moreover, much of this information is part of a shared 'pre-history' between doctor and patient, as are routines and action practices that both will rely on. This holds true for medical specialists treating long-term illnesses just as well as for general practitioners who may have seen a patient with changing ailments over the years.

These two broad types are further subdivided in research on medical encounters into at least four types of doctor-patient communication according to their *overall purposes* (Bührig and Meyer 2015; Löning 2001; Rehbein and Löning 1995):

a. anamnestic medical interview (see Bührig and Meyer 2009),
b. informed consent (see Bührig and Meyer 2015: 307; Meyer 2004),
c. delivery of diagnosis (with specific subtype of "bad news delivery", see Bührig and Meyer 2015: 308),
d. counselling (see Hartog 2006; Rehbein 2020).

In this subdivision, type (a) is primarily a first encounter, aiming at diagnosis, while types (b) to (d) represent follow-up encounters in the process of treating an illness. They aim at decision-making regarding further diagnostic and/or therapeutic procedures, as well as securing the patient's compliance and adherence to therapy. Type (d), namely counselling, may occur in particular when a serious illness is detected and a decision needs to be taken, in preventive healthcare, or if the patient brings up a subject of her/his own concern during a check-up. Counselling may actually take place within all kinds of DPC shortly before the closure of the encounter, especially if a patient makes use of a "final-concern sequence" in order to discuss "previously unmentioned mentionables" (White 2015: 175–177, 183–185).

Knowledge of the discourse types' general structure and overall purposes can be assumed to be part and parcel of the doctor's background, but not necessarily of the interpreter's. Since discourse structures typical of DPC are an integral part of a doctor's knowledge set, they naturally co-determine her/his chairing role throughout the encounter.

3.2 Internal Structures of DPC

Finally, discourse types are internally structured, again in accordance with the overall goals and purposes to be achieved. Looking at the only slight differences in category labelling by various authors, it becomes clear that the internal structure of a DPC encounter is a rather standard one in this institutional context, and it is fair to assume that it has been learned and internalized by the medical staff for DPC application.

The following purposes are linked to the standard structure of DPC by functional phases, as sketched out in Table 1:

Table 1 Internal structure of doctor-patient encounters

Valero-Garcés (2007)	Dubslaff and Martinsen (2007)	Pittarello (2012)
Initial greetings	Opening	Opening
Enunciation of problems	Medical history	Complaint
	Examination	Examination or test
Evaluation and discussion of the patient's condition	Diagnosis	Diagnosis
Discussion and prescription of the + treatments and/or check-ups	Consultation/ medical advice	Treatment or advice
Farewells		Closing

(1) *Opening*: introduces the purpose of the DPC at hand, including announcements preparing the patient for the imminent course of action to be taken, and serves to establish 'rapport' (Spencer-Oatey 2013; Dahm and Yates 2020) between doctor and patient;
(2) *Enunciation of problems*: establishes the medical history ('anamnesis', esp. in initial medical interviews), serves as stock-taking of the patient's current condition in order to create a basis for diagnostic evaluation; questions are used in particular to trigger verbalizations of perceived ailments on the patient's part in order to enable the doctor to interpret them in medical terms (Bührig and Meyer 2009: 189–191);
(3) *Evaluation and discussion* of the patient's condition (physical examination, diagnostic procedures): serves to establish a diagnosis and/or need of transfer to a specialist for further evaluation;
(4) *Discussion and prescription of treatment and/or check-ups, consultation and medical advice* (problem-solving, decision and treatment suggestion): serves to encourage patient compliance and adherence to therapeutic proposals, taking into account the patient's needs for counselling, support and further information;
(5) *Closing* (often preceded by an agreement regarding further appointments): closes the current speech situation while establishing rapport in order to maintain the joint action system for future interaction and to secure compliance and treatment success, farewells.

These five functional phases of DPC reflect a series of speech actions organized in accordance with the medical experts' knowledge of institutionalized action patterns. According to Functional Pragmatics, they are characterized by specific sequences or concatenations of speech actions which guide the hearer through perception and reception, and trigger the post-history of the hearer's subsequent action (Redder 2008: 138, 155). As institutionalized action patterns, they are part of second-order knowledge and can be understood as macro structures for interaction on the part of the institutional agents, e.g. doctors and possibly other medical staff. They include verbal, paraverbal and non-verbal knowledge that is drawn on when carrying out medical encounters. For instance, speech action patterns of announcing, explaining or proposing an action plan within the medical encounter can be employed in order to actively involve a patient. Extract 1 from the data, below, illustrates how the *opening* phase of DPC can pose challenges for IDPC.

At an even deeper level, micro-structures of knowledge are at work below the level of speech action patterns. The small units that speech actions are composed of are linguistic devices called 'procedures'. They operate as "instruments through which the speaker makes the hearer do something", i.e. makes them focus their attention, call upon certain knowledge, modify their expectations, etc. (Redder 2008: 138–139). These procedures can be differentiated as belonging to five different functional areas, linguistic fields that are determined by general communicative purposes common to all languages (deictic field, symbol field, operative field, tinge field, incitement field, respectively; in detail see Redder 2008: 138–142). According to FP, cognitive/mental processes are triggered by language-specific linguistic procedures (deictic, symbolic, operative, expressive and incitive) which are part of these linguistic fields. Extract(s) 2 (a and b) from the data, below, illustrates how operative and deictic procedures in seemingly everyday expressions, e.g. *matrix constructions* such as "I think (that)" can pose challenges in the *closing* phase of DPC for IDPC. In DPC, matrix constructions are employed by doctors in order to make evaluative statements, aimed at triggering specific mental processing of the doctor's utterance on the part of the patient (see Example 2 below).

3.3 *Knowledge Shared by the Interpreter*

To what extent, though, do interpreters share this specialized institutional knowledge? Are they familiar with the respective internal (micro) and external (macro) structures and how these are expressed in dialogue? Knowledge of this kind allows insights firstly into how the conversations are embedded into the overarching institutional processes (Bührig et al. 2000), secondly, into their internal purposes as outlined in some detail above, and, thirdly, into the implications of the more subtle speech actions implemented by the doctors. These may include efforts to elicit metaphorical descriptions of pain or the targeted use of questioning strategies in order to preclude a specific diagnosis (Bührig 2009: 156f, 166; Bührig and Meyer 2009: 198–202; Rehbein 1993, 1994). A subsequent question is whether it is a lack of knowledge about such functions of specific wordings and questioning techniques in medical encounters that may explain findings of trained medical interpreters' performance being insufficient and impeding rather than supporting the IDPC (Bührig and Meyer 2004, 2009: 197). The assumption behind this question is that, from the cognitive perspective adopted here, there may be an unperceived mismatch in what is taken for common ground between medical staff in charge of an encounter and medical interpreters. The former is expected to follow a goal-oriented action plan based on a heightened awareness of internal and external (institutional) structures, the respective action patterns and their purposes. When interpreters do not share such knowledge, they may be unable to infer meaning as implied by the doctor or to judge the relevance of targeted phrases and expressions. As a consequence, strategic interpreter processing, such as anticipation, may be impeded, and misjudgement of the importance of (rendering) certain expressions used by the doctor may ensue. It has been found, for instance, that almost 90% of mitigating and rapport-building expressions, such as hedges or phatics, are left unrendered by medical interpreters in the corpus data we deal with in this paper (Albl-Mikasa et al. 2015). Similarly, the above-mentioned matrix constructions are often omitted by the interpreters (see Example 2 below). Our assumption is that they may be omitted because interpreters are unaware of the specific role these expressions play in the DPC action plan.

The potential functional problems are obvious: when interpreters do not know that the welcoming section at the beginning of an encounter serves to build rapport with the patient or that the following treatment discussion aims to establish patient compliance (as explained above), they are more likely to omit expressions chosen by the doctor for that very (but unrecognized) purpose (see Baraldi and Gavioli 2020: 40–44, for issues regarding compliance in interpreted and mediated healthcare with migrant patients; see Dahm and Yates 2020: 213–215, for a discussion of challenges in rapport-building among international doctors in English as an L2). Omitting speech actions designed by doctors to build rapport may jeopardize treatment success, because building rapport establishes trust, enables patients' active participation and works towards compliance. As indispensable features of patient-centred care that contribute to a well-functioning interpersonal relationship between doctor and patient and to the patient's recovery, their rendering in the patient's language is required—be it in IDPC or when the doctor uses an L2 (Baraldi and Gavioli 2020: 40–41; Dahm and Yates 2020: 210–213).

In the following, we will first describe the corpus data, methodological approach and overall results of ongoing analyses, before presenting and discussing two extracts from the data that illustrate the points made, using the functional-pragmatic notions of action patterns and procedures introduced above.

4 Data and Methodological Approach

From a methodological point of view, methods consisting of "recording, transcribing and analysing spontaneous spoken interaction" (Wadensjö 2001: 195–196) have largely been relied on under the DI paradigm. In order to gain an understanding of interpreters' subjective requirements, motives and goals, recordings of interpreted doctor-patient encounters would have to be complemented with retrospective interviews. In the IDPC encounters studied here, access to the interpreters after the recordings was not given. Instead, from a FP point of view, conclusions can be drawn from the speech actions themselves, since they are linked to and reflect underlying cognitive processes.

In analysing two extracts from the corpus described below, we will illustrate health professionals' speech action patterns and their interpreted renditions. From this, we will point to relevant assumptions and working hypotheses regarding knowledge-based processes which, in follow-up studies, can be empirically investigated using both product-based transcribed and process-oriented introspective data.

Our analysis is based on video-recorded data from authentic doctor-patient encounters from the larger-scale study "Interpreting in Medical Settings: Roles, Requirements and Responsibility", funded between 2010 and 2012 by the Swiss Commission for Technology and Innovation (CTI, or KTI in German, now Innosuisse). The corpus has also been referred to as KTI project data (Albl-Mikasa 2019 and elsewhere). The study was carried out by an interdisciplinary team of medical specialists from the University Hospital of Basel (Marina Sleptsova and colleagues) and interpreting studies/applied linguistics researchers from the Zurich University of Applied Sciences (ZHAW) (Gertrud Hofer and colleagues). The core of their empirical data consists of 19 authentic, interpreted conversations (14.42 h, 856 min) along with a broad, questionnaire-based survey regarding the role of interpreters as perceived by medical personnel as well as medical interpreters (Sleptsova et al. 2014). In the interpreted conversations, German- and Swiss-German-speaking doctors and healthcare personnel interacted with patients of Turkish and Albanian origin at the university hospitals of Basel and Zurich and the Inselspital Bern. The interpreters were medical interpreters employed by the hospitals or contracted through cantonal interpreter service providers. As outlined by Sleptsova et al. (2017: 1668), half of the interpreters underwent a qualification programme at their employing institutions, the other half obtained specific interpreter training. In Switzerland, the schemes under which such continuing education measures run usually involve two to four days of training, qualifying the interpreter to act as an "intercultural interpreter" in accordance with standards approved by the Swiss Federal Office of Public Health (FOPH). The encounters were video-recorded and transcribed using the transcription software EXMARaLDA. The Turkish and Albanian parts were translated and the translations double-checked. The original data were transcribed using literal standard orthography, employing standard interpunction to mark utterances and their basic illocutions (i.e. stating, asking etc.). For functional-pragmatic analyses, the excerpt data were re-transcribed according to the HIAT standard for linguistic functional-pragmatic transcription (Ehlich 1992; Rehbein et al. 2004). The HIAT standard allows for multimodal transcription and analyses because it uses so-called *scores*, similar to music transcription: each speaker is represented in their own *tier*, and multiple tiers can be added per speaker to transcribe their multimodal activities, such as gestures and movements. In addition, annotation and commentary tiers are used to capture translations and transcribers' observational comments. Special notation is used for pauses (•, for minimal, and ((1,2 s)) for pauses of 1 s or above), repairs (/) and abandoned speech actions (…).

As described in some detail in Albl-Mikasa (2019: 256), various analyses have been conducted on the transcribed data, ranging from general renditions-based and accuracy-geared analyses to more specific investigations of omitted institutional procedures, such as hedges and phatic expressions, or the consequences of a lack of domain-specific and institutional process-based knowledge. During these data processing and evaluation developments, FP-based analyses of the data have turned out to be particularly promising, because of the focus on knowledge structures reflecting action patterns, which can be accessed and reconstructed linguistically (for FP methodology, see Bührig, Fienemann and Schlickau 2020: 71–73; Rehbein 2020: 85–93, both on interpreted medical counselling). Updating the Heidelberg School's cognitive and pragmatic discourse model of interpreting by integrating insights from FP (see Sect. 2) makes it possible to link pragmatic speech action phenomena to the underlying mental structures (Ehlich and Rehbein, 1986; Redder 2008). From this perspective, knowledge of (speech) action patterns forms a strong basis upon which interpreters reconstruct and reproduce target language utterances from source language utterances. For healthcare settings, in particular, FP studies have highlighted how internalized action patterns related to institutional interaction processes guide doctor-patient communication and medical counselling (Bührig et al. 2020; Rehbein 1994, 2020, among others). This is because institutionalized action patterns have evolved with and are closely tied to specific linguistic forms and it is linguistic choices that trigger and steer specific action courses (Rehbein 1993; Rehbein and Löning 1995). If, in multilingual DPC constellations, they are not taken up in the interpreting process, the course of DPC may be affected (Bührig et al. 2000; Bührig 2009; Bührig and Meyer 2009, 2015; Rehbein 1994). The integration of FP thus allows us to analyse how interpreters render linguistic action patterns representing institutional routines typically followed by medical personnel in DPC (and ideally reproduced by the interpreters) and to investigate the effects of access to or lack of action-pattern-related knowledge structures.

It needs to be noted that earlier approaches (Tebble 2009, 2014) have emphasized the importance of interpreters developing an understanding of the nature and structure of speech events, the metalinguistic or organizational language used as part of doctors' strategies and of the discursive moves associated with individual words (such as *right, well now, good*, etc.). In her genre-based approach, Tebble (2009: 208) also touches upon the cognitive dimension of this functional view: "If you understand the genre of the speech event for which you are interpreting then you have in mind a schema, a frame or a structure for understanding where the consultation or interview is going". The difference between this Systemic Functional Linguistics approach and the Functional Pragmatics one applied here is that the former only allows for an integration of background knowledge about discourse structures and markers, whereas the latter renders accessible cognitive processing as reflected in speech action patterns and linguistic devices that have evolved and are associated with institutional routines.

5 Empirical Evidence of the Significance of (Un)shared Knowledge

The following discussion of two speech action sequences from our data is a continuation of the overall analysis process of that data. As outlined in Albl-Mikasa (2019: 252–253), after a classic rendition-based analysis using atlas.ti tagging (Sleptsova et al. 2015), project efforts revealed the apparent lack of purpose-oriented institutional background knowledge causing substantial omission of source speech items. This led on to FP-based analyses, which point not only to a lack of shared background knowledge in terms of second-order institutional knowledge, but also to the non-recognition of important speech action patterns directly associated with the above-mentioned knowledge structures typical of DPC (Albl-Mikasa and Hohenstein 2017; Albl-Mikasa 2019). This approach considers how (non-)understanding on the part of the interpreter comes about, regarding the given institutional set-up of an encounter, its specific speech routines, linguistic procedures and set phrases and expressions. Methodologically, it entails a reconstruction of reception processes on the hearer's part, i.e. the interpreter as the hearer who mentally processes the German utterances of the doctor, and the patient as the hearer mentally processing the utterances interpreted into their L1 (in our two examples below, Turkish).

The below analysis of two examples follows up on this approach in that it looks at FP-based 'procedures', i.e. purposefully chosen linguistic units that play an active role in supporting or realizing a (speech) action and help the speaker in making adaptations and changes to the hearer's mental reality and knowledge structures (see Ehlich 1985/2007; 1993/2007, with regard to DPC). While expressions with deictic procedures (e.g. *I, you, here, then, that*) serve to re-focus the hearer's attention on the speaker, objects, people, locations or points in time and space without being referred to by appellative (symbolic) devices, symbolic procedures instantiate "societally constituted knowledge complexes" (Redder 2008: 139) in the hearer's mental space, condensed into nouns, verbs or adjectives, for instance. Both deictic and symbolic procedures are instrumental in our first example, Extract 1, for realizing the opening sequence of an IDPC between a German-speaking female doctor, DocF1, and a Turkish-speaking female patient, PatF1T. The example illustrates how larger, 'macro' structures of interaction, such as the speech action pattern of announcing, get transformed in the interpreter's rendering, and create a hearer's process for PatF1T in Turkish that is substantially altered in comparison to that ensuing from the doctor's original speech actions.

In the second example, Extract(s) 2 (a and b), operative procedures are crucial to the doctor's assessment of the patient's prospects. Operative procedures are "devices that assist the hearer in processing the structure of an utterance with regard to the syntactic function of its constituents, its propositional content, and its status in terms of discursive expectations" (Redder 2008: 139). Determiners, conjunctions, connectives, particles, interrogatives, case and gender morphemes, and sentence intonation are operative procedures. The following analysis illustrates how a non-rendition on the interpreter's part of certain speech actions (in Extract 1) and of seemingly trivial routine (matrix) expressions (in Extracts 2a and b) may affect the course of the conversation and impede its goals and purposes. The first example is an elaborated version of our first, brief introduction of an FP-based cognitive-pragmatic approach to medical interpreting (Albl-Mikasa and Hohenstein 2017). The second example is introduced to complement the macro-structure analysis with a micro-structure analysis.

The extracts chosen illustrate how both macro- and micro-structures of DPC that pertain to the doctor's second-order institutional knowledge can lead to renderings in IDPC that can affect patient involvement and the patient's experience of DPC. Instances of both are pervasive in the corpus. Both extracts are taken from German-Turkish IDPC in Swiss hospitals (as described above), illustrating one opening (Extract 1) and one closing phase (Extracts 2a and b). Research on DPC has established that the opening and closing phases of DPC are important in creating rapport and involvement for patients. As indispensable parts of patient-centred care, rapport and involvement are known to help patients, particularly in the case of long-term illnesses. Both extracts are chosen from follow-up encounters relating to long-term illnesses, so the patient and doctor have an established pre-history the interpreter is no part of. In order to choose these from the corpus, an inspection of all data based on preceding analyses was carried out. Two aspects were recurring in the data, namely altered speech action patterns and the deletion of institutionally functional operative procedures in renderings, and both can be linked to second-order knowledge. Extracts 1 and 2 were chosen because of their relative compactness while offering complex insights into the aspects detailed above.

In analyzing the two examples, we followed analytical steps as described in Redder (2008: 142–143), for instance: The video- and/or audio-recorded data underwent computer-based transcription according to the HIAT standard, the constellation and the pre- and post-history of the interaction were noted down, and the discourse was explored for macro-structural units and divided into sections. The utterances were assessed and segmented according to illocutionary and procedural qualities, and the sections were paraphrased for an overall assessment of the course of action, speech actions, interactional 'loops' etc. Based on these steps, a detailed interpretative analysis was conducted for sections where illocutionary and propositional differences between the doctor's original utterances and their rendering in the patient's language were detectable. The chosen examples are illustrative of systematically detectable differences (1) between the speech action pattern(s) used by the doctor and the speech actions resulting from the interpreted renderings, and (2) between linguistic procedures used with a specific function in the DPC and renderings in the target language where seemingly similar procedures are employed that do not achieve the same functional result. Both are related to second-order knowledge the doctor has at her/his disposal as an institutional agent, which the interpreter as an outsider and non-agent in the medical institution (hospital) does not share.

5.1 *Extract 1: Knowledge of Speech Actions and Institutional Action Patterns*

Extract 1 represents an instance of IDPC between a Swiss-German female doctor (DocF1) who uses Standard German and a female Turkish patient (PatF1T) with little L2 German. The female interpreter (IntF1) with L1 Turkish and L2 German has a training background in intercultural interpreting as described above. The patient has been treated for multiple medical issues, notably cancer of the right kidney, paralysis and immobility problems (the patient previously had to use a wheelchair) as well as bladder inflammation. Bearing the patient's medical history in mind, the following example is typical of *follow-up encounters* in the case of long-term illness or chronic disease. Extract 1 starts right at the beginning of the encounter between DocF1 and PatF1T. The transcript uses the so-called *score* representation associated with the functional-pragmatic methodology to allow for a notation of several simultaneous speech events, non-verbal communication etc. (Redder 2008: 142; Ehlich 1993). The scores are labelled with numbers in square brackets at the top left of each score. Extract 1 comprises scores [1], [2] and [3] and provides a *tier* (line) for each speaker, labelled at the left-hand side of each score. The original verbal utterances of the doctor in German are given in the *tier* labelled "DocF1 [v]" with a translation into English in small font in the tier below that, labelled "DocF1 [TL]". The utterances made in part in German, and in part in Turkish by the patient are given in the tier labelled "PatF1T [v]" and their translation into English in a tier labelled "PatF1T [TL]" below that. In the same manner, the interpreter's utterances are given in tiers labelled "IntF1 [v]" and "IntF1 [TL]". Reference to utterances is made using the score numbers in square brackets (e.g. [1]) in addition to so-called *event numbers* counting the utterances from 1 to 8, shown in the upper horizontal frame tier of each score (grey background) (Fig. 4).

Extract 1: Opening phase of the IDPC (KTl-Nr.11424.1 PFES-ES_Vid1), 20 s. at min. 01:28.0–01:49.5.

The doctor DocF1's first speech action addresses the patient by name (score [1], 0). PatF1T answers immediately in German (score [1], 1). Her reaction as a hearer in German enables us to reconstruct her understanding: not only does she understand that much German, she actively assumes the role of a hearer in that speech action pattern and, in doing so, re-establishes the pre-existing joint action system between DocF1 and herself.

The doctor then follows up with three speech actions of announcing which serve to structure the course of action ahead and render it accessible to PatF1T. First (in score [1], 2), the doctor *announces* to the patient that the interaction is about to start, using two deictic procedures, "jetzt" ('now'), which in German serves to re-focus the hearer's attention to the actual speech situation in time and space, and "wir" ('we'), which directs the hearer's attention to the fact that a joint action including the hearer is to be expected. This announcement is not rendered in Turkish. It is possible that PatF1T understands on her own and that IntF1 assumes so. Only the

[1]

	0	1	2	3	4
DocF1 [v]	Frau D.		Jetzt fangen wir an.	Eem wir machen heute ne Kontrolle.	Und jetzt habe ich als
DocF1 [TL]	Ms D.		We are starting now.	Um we are going to do a check-up today.	And now I have a question first.
DocF1 [nv]	sits down				((points to fingers of PatF1T))
PatF1T [v]		Ja			
PatF1T [TL]		Yes			

[2]

		5	6
DocF1 [v]	erstes ne Frage.	Haben Sie Blut abgegeben für INR-Kontrolle?	
DocF1 [TL]		Did you give a blood sample for INR testing?	
DocF1 [nv]			
IntF1 [v]			Eee bugün sadece kontrol
IntF1 [TL]			Uhh today there will only be a check-up,

[3]

		7	8
PatF1T [v]		Nanay.	
PatF1T [TL]		No.	
PatF1T [nv]		((shakes her head))	
IntF1 [v]	yapacak, bu	kontroldan sonra sonuç alıcak.	Kan verdinizmi bügün?
IntF1 [TL]	after that	check-up there will be a result.	Did you give a blood sample today?

Fig. 4 Extract 1, speech action pattern of announcing

following two *announcements*, namely ‘Um we are going to do a check-up today’ (score [1], 3) and ‘And now I have a question first’ (in [1], 4), are rendered in Turkish by the interpreter. In the German utterance announcing the imminent check-up ([1], 3), DocF1 again uses the inclusive first-person plural deictic “wir” and an inclusive personal predicate (“are going to do”). In doing so, the doctor announces a joint action to be carried out and reinforces the action system established with the patient. In functional-pragmatic terms, announcements belong to a speech action pattern used in constellations where the hearer has no control over the imminent actions, aiming to render mentally accessible to the hearer a course of action planned by the speaker (Hohenstein 2005: 296–298; Rehbein 1981). As Bührig et al. (2020: 73) point out, an important function of announcing is to enable the hearer to take a decision with respect to the imminent action, which is not always the case in medical encounters. In other words, doctors’ announcements are intended to facilitate patients’ mental anticipation of the joint course of action and to enable them to comply in a speech situation where their range of control and scope of action are limited. From a German hearer’s perspective, an announcement can be processed to that effect. A rendering in Turkish needs to trigger the same kind of mental processes on the part of the hearer, PatF1T. The Turkish rendering “Eee, bugün sedece control yapacak” (scores [2–3], 6), which was translated as an impersonal construction, can actually be read as a third-person construction ‘Uhh today she will only do a check-up’. It produces an illocutionary force different from an announcement. By transforming the first-person deictic procedures to a third-person descriptive predicate, the joint action system is discontinued, the effect is that of *introducing* an action plan that has been decided on already and is only communicated to the hearer, PatF1T. The effect of using introductions is also discussed in Bührig et al. (2020: 73–75, 78), where a link is drawn to pre-prepared plans on the doctor’s part that tend to be executed with little consideration for shared decision-making and patient empowerment. What becomes clear from that perspective is that interpreted pattern shifts from announcing to introducing planned actions may lead to the disempowerment of the patient and to less patient-centred care.

In fact, the 'result' that the interpreter mentions ("sonra sonuç alıcak", 'then there will be a result' or 'then you will get a result', score [3], 6) has not been mentioned by the doctor and is not the purpose of the current interaction. As a symbol field expression, it instantiates "societally constituted knowledge complexes" for the hearer, and, in her rendering, IntF1 constructs and supplies a purposeful relation in her own right. In addition, she uses the mitigating expression "sadece" ('only') that serves to play down the planned action, making the purpose—i.e. checking up on the patient in the aftermath of cancer therapy—appear to be a trivial matter. Both added elements trigger cognitive processing on PatF1T's part in Turkish that differs substantially from the linguistic procedures at work in the German utterances.

Another transformation of DocF1's utterances comes about when she announces her question regarding the blood sample for INR testing before *actually posing* the question in her next utterance (scores [1–2], 4). More specifically, the doctor uses a temporal deictic procedure ("jetzt", 'now'), indicating that her question *precedes* the next step in the interaction and instilling an expectation in the patient of the course of action. The interpreter overrides that announcement by simply asking the question (score [3], 8). In functional-pragmatic terms, opening sections serve to prepare patients for the course of action to be expected during the DPC. The fact that the three announcements in Extract 1 ('We are starting now', 'Um we are going to do a check-up today' and 'And now I have a question first') do not contain any language- or terminology-related difficulties leads us to assume that the interpreter may have been unaware of the rapport-building and meta-discursive function of these opening speech actions. This may have been why her rendition deviated from the source language presentation and inadvertently transformed the speech actions' illocutionary force.

PatF1T's reaction to the doctor's question ('Did you give a blood sample for INR testing', score [2], 5) allows us to reconstruct that the patient understood and can relate to the use of the medical term "INR" since she reacts with a negation ("Nanay", 'no, not yet' in score [3], 7) with a small delay to the doctor's question. The interpreter, by contrast, omits the medical expression "INR testing" (score [2–3], 6 and 8), which suggests that she does not know the expression or the specific procedure it refers to. This, in turn, leads us to assume that the relevant institutional knowledge shared by the patient (semi-professional knowledge as a client of the institution, see above; Rehbein 2020: 90) and doctor (institutional knowledge of second-order, as an agent of the institution, see above) is not part of the interpreter's background knowledge. Moreover, in the case of a medical follow-up encounter, as is the case in Extract 1, announcements of the imminent course of action are linked to the pre-history shared between doctors and patients. INR testing is a routine PatF1T has undergone several times already and knows to be part of a check-up. Since interpreters are not always a party to this pre-history, this poses a challenge for interpreting in any follow-up IDPC. It may affect the interpreter's mental participation in the doctor's action plan and prevent the rapport-building effect of an announcement's illocutionary force (i.e. goals and purpose of the utterance).

Extract (1) is an illustration of what appears to be cognitive non-processing on the interpreter's part of action pattern knowledge related to the standard structure of doctor-patient interaction. Substantial changes to the propositional build-up and to the doctor's speech actions may have resulted from the interpreter's lack of awareness of the institutionalized function of the *action pattern* of announcing. There are, of course, other possible reasons apart from non-recognition of the speech action pattern, such as cognitive overload. An explanation may be that the interpreter may not have understood the purpose of the current interactional phase, which is to set the goals of the DPC at hand, prepare the patient by making announcements for the imminent course of action to be taken and establish rapport. The crucial insight from Extract 1, however, is that even at the very beginning and with seemingly simple and short units of speech, substantial modifications may occur in the renditions with adverse effects on the doctor's and patient's joint action system, altering rapport-building and mutual understanding in the communicative action that is taking shape. Speech action patterns are socially *and* cognitively developed structures. When cast into utterances as part of linguistic interaction within institutional processes, they shed light on the underlying cognitive processes. Awareness of such action patterns related to the standard structure of doctor-patient interaction may help the interpreter to cognitively process and interpret the goals and purposes relevant to the institutional context.

5.2 Extract(s) 2 (A and B): Matrix Constructions and Mental Processing Below the Level of Pattern Knowledge

The following second example is incorporated here to illustrate how *cognitive processing* at the level of linguistic micro-structures, below the level of speech action patterns, may be affected in the DPC interpreting process. To this end, three matrix constructions are looked at more closely. Matrix constructions are complex syntactic structures that subordinate and embed an utterance or sentence as a partial structure by means of a complementizer, e.g. "dass"/ "that" in German/English. While the embedded part is a fully-fledged propositional act, the illocutionary force is carried by the matrix construction. By making use of verba sentiendi (e.g. "Ich denke, dass"/ "I think that", Hohenstein 2004; 2007: 419–424) for instance, the matrix construction serves to relate assessments, evaluations and claims. Experts, such as doctors, can use matrix constructions to superimpose a note of authority judgement, assertion or conviction on the fact conveyed in the embedded part. By supplementing the factual information in the embedded clause with her or his expert knowledge and opinion, a doctor is able to render utterances like "I think your healing prospects are very good" more reassuring. Matrix constructions belong to a class of linguistic expressions that are analyzed as 'stance', 'hedges' or 'complement constructions'. While hedges may tone down doctors' statements, e.g. for safeguarding purposes ("Your healing prospects are very good" vs "As far as can be said at this point, your healing prospects are very good"), matrix constructions of thinking and believing may serve to underpin a statement with a doctor's expert positioning ("I think that your healing prospects are very good"). They can help patient's process medical information from the doctor's expert knowledge in relation to their own knowledge structures. Such positioning by the doctor creates "interaction coherence" and a synchronization of the speaker's and the hearer's mental processes in the sense that the doctor invites the patient to share her/his assessment and helps the patient to relate to it (Hohenstein 2004: 330; Rehbein 2007: 419–424, 429–431).

As follows from the analysis of Extract(s) 2 (a and b) below, three German matrix constructions used in the doctor's assessment of the patient's healing prospects are rendered in the process of interpreting into Turkish in a way that changes the doctor's utterances at both the propositional and illocutionary level.

This second IDPC extract is taken from a follow-up encounter between a Swiss-German male doctor (DocM1) and a female Turkish patient (PatF2T). It is interpreted by another female, trained intercultural community interpreter (IntF2) with L1 Turkish and L2 German. The patient has undergone surgery and chemotherapy to treat breast cancer, is currently receiving radiotherapy and has severe pains in her left side. The extract is from the final phase of the consultation when DocM1 starts closing by asking the patient whether she has any further questions. The patient explains that, in order to find her peace again, she needs to know that no cancer is left in her body. Extracts 2a and b represent the doctor's answer and its rendition in Turkish by the interpreter.

Extract 2a: Closing phase of the DPC (KTl-Nr.11424.1 PFES-ES_Vid2), score frame 328, min. 27:12.2. The transcript provides the utterances in German and Turkish of each speaker in large font (DocM1 [v]; IntF2 [v]) with an English gloss in smaller font below (DocM1 [TL]; IntF2 [TL]). For further explanation of the transcript standard etc., see Extract 1, above.

In Extract 2a (see Fig. 5), the doctor gives an expert opinion of the patient's healing prospects. The overall tenor of DocM1's utterances from scores [1] to [5] is that of positively reassuring the patient of her benign prospects and, at the same time, making sure not to make false promises. The mitigations in scores [2], 4–6 and [3–4], 6–7 serve this latter purpose, but are not rendered in the Turkish interpretation, as can be seen in Extract 2b (see Fig. 6). Following the patient's request for clarification regarding her healing prospects, DocM1 uses three *matrix constructions* 'I think', 'the chances are excellent that' and 'the chance is very good that' (score [1], 1–3, and score [4], 8–9) to convey the requested propositional information. The 'I think' construction is not simply a subjective stance or personal judgement. Pragmatically speaking, as both the deictic centre and the subject of that construction, DocM1 emphasizes his *expert perspective* as a medical doctor and as an agent within the medical institution. The assertive illocutionary force of the matrix construction 'I think' turns the complete utterance into an *assessment*. Cognitively speaking, the construction facilitates a mental process on the hearer's part (the patient, in L1 DPC,

	0 1	2	3
[nr]	score 328/ 663 [27:12.2]		665 [27:15.9]
DocM1 [v]	Hm̀hm̀ ich denke,	die Chancen sind hervorragend,	dass kein Krebs mehr da ist. ‿
DocM1 [TL]	Well, I think	the chances are excellent	that there is no more cancer.

[2]

	4	5	6
[nr]	666 [27:17.9]		667 [27:21.6]
DocM1 [v]	Aber man muss immer sagen,	wir können die Zukunft nicht sicher vorhersagen. ‿	Ich kann
DocM1 [TL]	But one always needs to say,	we cannot predict the future exactly.	I cannot

[3]

		7
[nr]		
DocM1 [v]	Ihnen das nicht versprechen und schwören,	das ist/ das gibt immer natürlich
DocM1 [TL]	promise you and swear it to you,	that is/ there are always of course surprises in life.

[4]

		8	9
[nr]		668 [27:27.4]	
DocM1 [v]	Überraschungen im Leben.	Aber die Chance ist sehr gut,	dass wir alles wegbekommen
DocM1 [TL]		But the chance is very good	that we could erase it all

[5]

	10	11	12
[nr]		669 [27:34.0]	670
DocM1 [v]	haben mit der Chemotherapie, der Strahlentherapie, der	Operation, alles zusammen.	
DocM1 [TL]	with the help of the chemotherapy, the radiotherapy, the	operation, all together.	
IntF2 [v]		yani şansımız diyo büyük.	• •
IntF2 [TL]		Actually our chances, he says, are good.	• •

Fig. 5 Extract 2a: Matrix constructions in doctor's utterance

the interpreter in IDPC), giving them access to the proposition in terms of a qualified expert assessment instead of a simple statement. In the Turkish rendition, which replaces the doctor's stance 'I think' with 'he says', both aspects, that the doctor is *sharing his opinion* in his capacity as an expert, and that, from this position, he makes an *expert assessment* of the patient's outcome, is lost.

The main clause 'the chances are excellent' states a positive evaluation of the patient's outcome; however, by following it up with "that" the doctor turns it into a second matrix construction. He embeds into this construction 'there is no more cancer', rephrasing parts of what the patient had verbalized before: her doubts about not having any more cancer cells in her body. This embedded *factual proposition* links up the doctor's expert medical perspective (verbalized in the matrix construction) with the patient's perspective (taken up in the embedded subordinate proposition), establishing '*interaction coherence*' as outlined above.

The third matrix construction ('the chance is very good that') used by the doctor in [4], 8–9 again states a positive evaluation of the patient's outcome. The embedded proposition assumes a personal, inclusive perspective by using the (plural) speaker deictic "wir" ('we could erase it all [...]'). Here, too, the two perspectives are linked, aiming at interaction coherence: making the cognitive processing of medical facts in the form of an expert assessment accessible and achieving an assertive positive illocution. These effects are lost in the interpretation. By using reported speech ('he says'), the interpreter IntF2 in score [5], utterance 11, gives an *account of the doctor's*

[5]

	10	11	12
[nr]		*669 [27:34.0]*	*670*
DocM1 [v]	haben mit der Chemotherapie, der Strahlentherapie, der	Operation, alles zusammen.	
DocM1 [TL]	with the help of the chemotherapy, the radiotherapy, the	operation, all together.	
IntF2 [v]		yani şansımız diyo büyük.	• •
IntF2 [TL]		Actually our chances, he says, are good.	• •

[6]

	13	14	15
[nr]	*[27:34.4] 671 [27:36.4]*		*672 [27:41.3]*
IntF2 [v]	yani şansımız çok büyük, em	ameliyatla kemother/ em kemoterapiyle	ışın
IntF2 [TL]	actually our chances are very good, um	with the operation, the chemother/ um chemotherapy	and radiotherapy,

[7]

		16	17	18
[nr]				*673 [27:47.1]*
IntF2 [v]	tedavisinle,	yani şansımız	çok çok büyük birşey kalmadığına dair,	ama tabi gelecekte hiç
IntF2 [TL]		actually the chances	are very, very good that nothing remains,	but for the future we cannot say

[8]

		19
[nr]		*674 [27:53.9]*
PatF2T [v]		Birde kendilerinin gene bana söylediğine
PatF2T [TL]		And plus that all the physicians told me again
IntF2 [v]	birşey söyliyemeyiz, yani ne çıkar ne olur bunu.	
IntF2 [TL]	what will become of it, what will happen from it.	

Fig. 6 Extract 2b: Interpreter's rendition of three matrix constructions

speech action instead of expressing an expert assessment. Instances of changes in role behaviour or perspective (i.e. the interpreter's adopting the third person singular) or reporting (i.e. not presenting the speaker directly) have been observed repeatedly in the analysis of recorded IDPC (e.g. Johnen and Meyer 2007). What makes the cognitive-pragmatic perspective taken here particularly interesting is that it illustrates the deeper level of meaning that patients miss out on when interpreters do not adhere to the institutionalized discourse structures used by healthcare professionals, ultimately with the risk of compromising the therapeutic outcome.

The interpreter's utterances in scores [5], 11 and [6], 13–15 fail to reproduce *an equivalent of the matrix constructions*. The matrix ('actually the chances are very very large that') and factual statement ('nothing remains') do not enable the patient to adjust her own knowledge structures according to the doctor's guidance. As can be seen from the following analysis, interaction coherence is not secured. Even though the Turkish utterance [7]-[8], 18 ('but for the future, we cannot say what will become of it, what will happen from it') picks up on the adversative structure ("ama", 'but') and propositional reference to the 'future', the illocution rendered by the interpreter in scores [5] to [8] differs substantially from the doctor's message. Instead of conveying the optimistic outlook inherent in the doctor's expert assessment, it *tones down* the patient's prospects. In part, this is due to the modals 'actually' and 'very' and referring to 'good' instead of 'excellent' chances, symbol field procedures triggering different assessments. From the patient's reaction following this rendition, it becomes clear that her peace of mind was not restored: instead, she launches an account of how several physicians had actually discouraged her with regard to her healing (and survival) prospects.

From the above analysis, it becomes clear that linguistic micro-structures like matrix constructions represent and trigger goal-oriented mental processes. The reproduction of these constructions is therefore paramount if the intended cognitive processes are to be initiated in the hearer's mind and if interactional coherence is to be established. From the cognitive-pragmatic perspective taken here, one possible explanation for the alterations to the source utterances is that this deeper dimension of language use in DPC has not been understood by the interpreter and that the associated processes have not been activated in her mind while reproducing the Turkish utterances. If so, interpreters would need to be aware of the cognitive and pragmatic dimensions of these constructions systematically used in DPC in order to be able to render the goal-oriented mental processes accessible to patients' information processing in IDPC.

6 Conclusion

This paper is a continuation of efforts to usher in a cognitive turn in community interpreting studies (see Tiselius and Albl-Mikasa 2019). The exclusive focus on an interactive sociolinguistic perspective within the DI paradigm has its roots in Wadensjö's 1998 exclusion of the cognitive dimension. The consequent focus in community interpreting studies on role behaviour, turn management and communicative interaction has long dominated investigations of medical interpreting too. It is, however, in this field in particular that this approach has turned out to be reductionist. This is, in fact, one of the outcomes of the analyses of the Swiss Basel University Hospital/Zurich University of Applied Sciences corpus project (see Albl-Mikasa 2019), which inductively uncovered the importance of shared knowledge among the participants of doctor-patient encounters serving as an inferential basis for the fulfilment of societal functions through purpose-oriented discourse. A befitting framework for community interpreting is therefore seen in the Heidelberg School's cognitive-pragmatic discourse model of interpreting. Updated with insights from Functional Pragmatics, it makes it possible to describe community (including medical) interpreting as what it is, namely a socially *and* cognitively situated activity (Albl-Mikasa 2019, 2020).

This paper follows up on the authors' earlier chapter (Albl-Mikasa and Hohenstein 2017) by demonstrating the role knowledge plays in IDPC at higher (e.g. schemata about institutional processes) and lower (linguistic micro-structures) levels. It can be shown that a lack of understanding of the goal-oriented processes represented and triggered by micro-structures (such as matrix constructions) or macro-level speech action patterns (such as making announcements) adversely affects DPC interpreting. It is concluded that an understanding of these deeper dimensions of institutional knowledge and related language use may play a considerable role in processing the interactional complexity underlying any DPC and may be a prerequisite for helping doctors to follow through with their action plans, goals and purposes.

Interpreting being an act of pragmatic cognitive discourse processing, the interpreters' comprehension and production processes depend heavily on various types of linguistic and non-linguistic knowledge. Especially in settings like institutionalized medical interpreting in hospitals, a wide range of super- and subordinated knowledge types influence the interpreters' processing and performance: knowledge of larger institutional processes, of external and internal structures of discourse events (e.g. doctor-patient encounters), of specific related action patterns as well as of linguistic devices, such as hedges, phatic expressions and matrix constructions. FP-based analyses highlight not only the importance of sharing such knowledge structures, but how application of such knowledge becomes linguistic and non-linguistic discursive action. FP concepts, such as procedures and action patterns, if shared by the interpreter, enable institutional action processes to be carried through. Medical interpreting thus goes way beyond coordinating turns and conveying conversational snippets. To the extent that interpreters share these knowledge structures down to the level of expressions and lexical constructions, they enact institutional processes. The full scope of interpreters' action becomes apparent only through an integral view of the interactive, social and cognitive dimensions.

References

Albl-Mikasa, M. 2007. *Notationssprache und Notizentext. Ein kognitiv-linguistisches Modell für das Konsekutivdolmetschen.* Narr.

Albl-Mikasa, M. 2014. Receptivism. An intertraditional approach to intuition in interpreter and translator competence. In L.N. Zybatow, and M. Ustaszewski (Eds.), *Bausteine translatorischer Kompetenz oder was macht Übersetzer und Dolmetscher zu Profis. Innsbrucker Ringvorlesungen zur Translationswissenschaft VII* (pp. 51–81). Peter Lang.

Albl-Mikasa, M. 2019. Acting upon background of understanding rather than role: Shifting the focus from the interactional to the inferential dimension of (medical) dialogue interpreting. *Translation, Cognition and Behavior* 2 (2): 241–262. https://doi.org/10.1075/tcb.00028.alb.

Albl-Mikasa, M. 2020. Interpreters' roles and responsibilities. In E. Angelone, M. Ehrensberger-Dow, and G. Massey (Eds.), The Bloomsbury companion to language industry studies (pp. 91–114). Bloomsbury. https://doi.org/10.5040/9781350024960.0009.

Albl-Mikasa, M., and Hohenstein, C. 2017. Cognition in community interpreting: The influence of interpreters' knowledge of doctor-patient interaction. In D. Perrin, and U. Kleinberger (Eds.), *Doing applied linguistics: Enabling transdisciplinary communication* (pp. 130–138). De Gruyter. https://doi.org/10.1515/9783110496604-016.

Albl-Mikasa, M., Glatz, E., Hofer, G., and Sleptsova, M. 2015. Caution and compliance in medical encounters. Non-interpretation of hedges and phatic tokens. *Translation and Interpreting*, 7 (2): 76–89. https://doi.org/10.12807/ti.107203.2015.a06.

Angelelli, C. 2004. *Medical interpreting and cross-cultural communication.* Cambridge University Press.

Bancroft, M.A. 2015. Community interpreting: A profession rooted in social justice. In *The Routledge handbook of interpreting*, ed. H. Mikkelson and R. Jourdenais, 217–235. Routledge.

Baraldi, C., and Gavioli, L. 2020. Patients' initiatives and the achievement of medical compliance in talk with migrant patients and with(out) interpreting aid. In C. Hohenstein, and M. Lévy-Tödter (Eds.), *Multilingual healthcare. A global view on communicative challenges* (pp. 39–63). Springer Gabler. https://doi.org/10.1007/978-3-658-27120-6_3.

Bot, H. 2003. The myth of the uninvolved interpreter interpreting in mental health and the development of a three-person psychology. In L. Brunette, G.L. Bastin, I. Hemlin, and H. Clarke (Eds.), *The Critical Link 3: Interpreters in the community. Selected papers from the Third International Conference on Interpreting in Legal, Health and Social Service Settings, Montréal, Quebec, Canada 22–26 May 2001* (pp. 27–35). John Benjamins.
Braun, S. 2004. Kommunikation unter widrigen Umständen. Einsprachige und gedolmetschte Kommunikation in der Videokonferenz. *Target*, 20 (1): 176–180.
Braun, S., and Kohn, K. 2012. Towards a pedagogic corpus approach to business and community interpreter training. In B. Ahrens, M. Albl-Mikasa, and C. Sasse (Eds.), *Dolmetschqualität in Praxis, Lehre und Forschung. Festschrift für Sylvia Kalina* (pp. 185–204). Narr.
Brown, G., and G. Yule. 1983. *Discourse analysis*. Cambridge University Press.
Bührig, K. 2005. Speech action patterns" and "discourse types. *Folia Linguistica* 39 (1–2): 143–171. https://doi.org/10.1515/flin.2005.39.1-2.143.
Bührig, K. 2009. Interpreting in hospitals. Starting points for cultural actions in institutionalized communication. In K. Bührig, J. House, and J.D. ten Thije (Eds.), *Translational action and intercultural communication* (pp. 151–174). St. Jerome Publishing.
Bührig, K., Durlanık, L., and Meyer, B. 2000. *Arzt-Patienten-Kommunikation im Krankenhaus. Konstitutive Handlungseinheiten, institutionelle Handlungslinien*. Universität Hamburg, Sonderforschungsbereich Mehrsprachigkeit.
Bührig, K., and Meyer, B. 2004. Ad-hoc-interpreting and the achievement of communicative purposes in doctor-patient-communication. In J. House, and J. Rehbein (Eds.), *Multilingual Communication* (pp. 43–62). John Benjamins. https://doi.org/10.1075/hsm.3.04buh.
Bührig, K., and Meyer, B. 2009. Gespräche zwischen Patienten und Ärzten. Ein- und mehrsprachige Anamnesen im Krankenhaus. In N. Klusen, A. Fließgarten, and T. Nebling (Eds.), *Informiert und selbstbestimmt. Der mündige Bürger als mündiger Patient* (pp. 189–205). Nomos. https://doi.org/10.1075/hsm.3.04buh.
Bührig, K., Fienemann, J., and Schlickau, S. 2020. On certain characteristics of 'Diabetes Consultations'. In C. Hohenstein, and M. Lévy-Tödter (Eds.), *Multilingual healthcare. A global view on communicative challenges* (pp. 65–82). Springer Gabler. https://doi.org/10.1007/978-3-658-27120-6_4.
Bührig, K., and B. Meyer. 2013. Transfer is not a one-way street: Insights in ad-hoc interpreting in German hospitals. In *Transferring linguistic know-how into institutional practice*, ed. K. Bührig and B. Meyer, 137–150. John Benjamins.
Bührig, K., and B. Meyer. 2015. Gespräche mit MigrantInnen. In *Handbuch Sprache in der Medizin*, ed. A. Busch and T. Spranz-Fogasy, 300–316. de Gruyter.
Creeze, I. 2013. Introduction to healthcare for interpreters and translators. *John Benjamins*. https://doi.org/10.1075/z.181.
Dahm, Maria R., and Yates, L. 2020. Rapport, empathy and professional identity: Some challenges for international medical graduates speaking English as a second or foreign language. In C. Hohenstein, and M. Lévy-Tödter (Eds.), *Multilingual healthcare. A global view on communicative challenges* (pp. 209–234). Springer Gabler. https://doi.org/10.1007/978-3-658-27120-6_9.
Dubslaff, F., and Martinsen, B. 2007. Exploring untrained interpreters' use of direct versus indirect speech. In F. Pöchhacker, and M. Shlesinger (Eds.), *Healthcare interpreting* (pp. 53–76). John Benjamins Publishing Company. https://doi.org/10.1075/bct.9.06dub.
Ehlich, K. 1985/2007. The Language of Pain. Reprinted 2007 in K. Ehlich (Ed.), *Sprache und sprachliches Handeln*, Bd. 3, I 6 (pp. 243–254). Walter de Gruyter.
Ehlich, K. 1992. HIAT—A transcription system for discourse data. In *Talking data: Transcription and coding in discourse research*, ed. J.A. Edwards and M.D. Lampert, 123–148. Erlbaum.
Ehlich, K. 1993/2007. Sprachliche Prozeduren in der Arzt-Patienten-Kommunikation. Reprinted in K. Ehlich (Ed.), *Sprache und sprachliches Handeln*, Bd. 3, I 7 (pp. 255–279). Walter de Gruyter.
Ehlich, K., and Rehbein, J. 1986. *Muster und Institution*. Narr.

Englund Dimitrova, B., and Tiselius, E. 2016. Cognitive aspects of community interpreting. Towards a process model. In R. Muñoz Martín (Ed.), *Reembedding translation process research* (pp. 195–214). John Benjamins. https://doi.org/10.1075/btl.128.10eng.
Hartog, J. 1994. Die Methode des Zentralen Beziehungs-Konflikts-Themas (ZBKT): Eine linguistische Kritik. In *Medizinische Kommunikation, Diskurspraxis, Diskursethik, Diskursanalyse*, ed. A. Redder and I. Wiese, 306–326. Westdeutscher Verlag.
Hartog, J. 2006. Beyond 'misunderstandings' and 'cultural stereotypes'. Analysing intercultural communication. In K. Bührig, and J.D. ten Thije (Eds.), *Beyond misunderstanding. The linguistic reconstruction of intercultural discourse* (pp. 175–188). John Benjamins.
Hervais-Adelman, A., B. Moser-Mercer, and N. Golestani. 2015. Brain functional plasticity associated with the emergence of expertise in extreme language control. *NeuroImage* 114: 264–274. https://doi.org/10.1016/j.neuroimage.2015.03.072.
Hohenstein, C. 2004. A comparative analysis of Japanese and German complement constructions with matrix verbs of thinking and believing - *to omou* and *ich glaub(e)*. In *Multilingual communication*, ed. J. House and J. Rehbein, 303–341. Benjamins.
Hohenstein, C. 2005. Interactional expectations and linguistic knowledge in academic expert discourse (Japanese/German). *International Journal of the Sociology of Language* 175 (176): 285–306.
Hurtado Albir, A., and F. Alves. 2009. Translation as a cognitive activity. In *The Routledge companion to translation studies*, ed. J. Munday, 54–73. Routledge.
Johnen, T., and Meyer, B. 2007. Between connectivity and modality: Reported speech in interpreter-mediated doctor-patient communication. In J. Rehbein, C. Hohenstein, and L. Pietsch (Eds.), *Connectivity in grammar an discourse* (pp. 395–417). Benjamins. https://doi.org/10.1075/hsm.5.22joh.
Kalina, S. 1998. *Strategische Prozesse beim Dolmetschen. Theoretische Grundlagen, empirische Fallstudien, didaktische Konsequenzen.* Narr.
Kohn, K. 2011. English as a lingua franca and the standard English misunderstanding. In A. De Houwer, and A. Wilton (Eds.), *English in Europe today. Sociocultural and educational perspectives* (pp. 72–94). John Benjamins. https://doi.org/10.1075/aals.8.06koh.
Kohn, K., and S. Kalina. 1996. The strategic dimension of interpreting. *Meta* 61 (1): 118–138.
Löning, P. 1994. Versprachlichung von Wissenstrukturen bei Patienten. In *Medizinische Kommunikation: Diskurspraxis, Diskursethik, Diskursanalyse*, ed. A. Redder and I. Wiese, 97–111. Westdeutscher Verlag.
Löning, P. 2001. Gespräche in der Medizin. In K. Brinker, G. Antos, W. Heinemann, and S. F. Sager (Eds.), *Text- und Gesprächslinguistik. Ein internationales Handbuch zeitgenössischer Forschung* (pp. 1576–1588). de Gruyter. https://doi.org/10.1515/9783110169188.2.22.1576.
Martínez-Gómez, A. 2015. Non-professional interpreters. In *The Routledge handbook of interpreting*, ed. H. Mikkelson and R. Jourdenais, 417–431. Routledge.
Meyer, B. 2004. *Dolmetschen im medizinischen Aufklärungsgespräch: Eine diskursanalytische Untersuchung zur Wissensvermittlung im mehrsprachigen Krankenhaus.* Waxmann.
Ozolins, U. 2015. Ethics and the role of the interpreter. In *The Routledge handbook of interpreting*, ed. H. Mikkelson and R. Jourdenais, 319–336. Routledge.
Pittarello, S. 2012. Medical terminology circulation and interactional organisation in interpreter-mediated medical encounters. *Linguistica Antverpiensia New Series, Themes in Translation Studies*, 11: 113–131. https://doi.org/10.52034/lanstts.v11i.299.
Pöchhacker, F. 2012. Qualität, die man versteht: Ein funktional-kognitiver Ansatz. In B. Ahrens, M. Albl-Mikasa, and C. Sasse (Eds.), *Dolmetschqualität in Praxis, Lehre und Forschung. Festschrift für Sylvia Kalina* (pp. 19–31). Narr.
Pöchhacker, F. 2015. Evolution of interpreting research. In *The Routledge handbook of interpreting*, ed. H. Mikkelson and R. Jourdenais, 62–76. Routledge.
Redder, A. 2008. Functional Pragmatics. In G. Antos, and E. Ventola (Eds.), *Handbook of interpersonal communication* (pp. 133–178). de Gruyter. https://doi.org/10.1515/9783110211399.1.133.

Rehbein, J. 1981. Announcing - On formulating plans. In *Conversational Routine*, ed. F. Coulmas, 215–258. Mouton.
Rehbein, J. 1993. Ärztliches Fragen. Analysen zu einem interdisziplinären Problem. In P. Löning, and J. Rehbein (Eds.), *Arzt-Patienten-Kommunikation. Analysen zu interdisziplinären Problemen des medizinischen Diskurses* (pp. 311–363). de Gruyter.
Rehbein, J. 1994. Rejective proposals: Semi-professional speech and clients' varieties in intercultural doctor-patient communication. *Multilingua* 13 (2): 83–130.
Rehbein, J. 2007. Matrix constructions. In J. Rehbein, C. Hohenstein, and L. Pietsch (Eds.), *Connectivity in grammar and discourse* (pp. 419–447). John Benjamins. https://doi.org/10.1075/hsm.5.23reh.
Rehbein, J. 2020. Multilingual counselling in preventive healthcare. In C. Hohenstein, and M. Lévy-Tödter (Eds.), *Multilingual healthcare. A global view on communicative challenges* (pp. 83–131). Springer Gabler. https://doi.org/10.1007/978-3-658-27120-6_5.
Rehbein, J., and P. Löning. 1995. *Sprachliche Verständigungsprozesse in der Arzt-Patienten-Kommunikation: Linguistische Untersuchung von Gesprächen in der Facharzt-Praxis*. Germanisches Seminar: Universität Hamburg.
Rehbein, J., Schmidt, T., Meyer, B., Watzke, F., and Herkenrath, A. 2004. *Handbuch für das computergestützte Transkribieren nach HIAT*. Arbeiten zur Mehrsprachigkeit Folge B, 56 (2004). Hamburg: Universität Hamburg, Sonderforschungsbereich 538 Mehrsprachigkeit. https://exmaralda.org/de/hiat/.
Rosenberg, E., R. Seller, and Y. Leanza. 2008. Through interpreters' eyes: Comparing roles of professional and family interpreters. *Patient Education and Counseling* 70: 87–93. https://doi.org/10.1016/j.pec.2007.09.015.
Shiffrin, D. 1994. *Approaches to Discourse*. Blackwell.
Sleptsova, M., G. Hofer, N. Morina, and W. Langewitz. 2014. The role of the health care interpreter in a clinical setting—A narrative review. *Community Health Nursing* 31 (3): 167–184. https://doi.org/10.1080/07370016.2014.926682.
Sleptsova, M., G. Hofer, E. Marcel, P. Grossman, N. Morina, M. Schick, M.L. Daly, I. Weber, O. Kocagöncü, and W.A. Langewitz. 2015. Wie verstehen Dolmetscher ihre Rolle in medizinischen Konsultationen und wie verhalten sie sich konkret in der Praxis? *Psychotherapie, Psychosomatik, Medizinische Psychologie* 65 (9–10): 363–369. https://doi.org/10.1055/s-0035-1554691.
Sleptsova, M., H. Weber, A.C. Schöpf, M. Nübling, N. Morina, G. Hofer, and W. Langewitz. 2017. Using interpreters in medical consultations: What is said and what is translated—A descriptive analysis using RIAS. *Patient Education and Counseling* 100: 1667–1671. https://doi.org/10.1016/j.pec.2017.03.023.
Spencer-Oatey, H. 2013. Relating at Work: Facets, dialectics and face. *Journal of Pragmatics* 58: 121–137. https://doi.org/10.1016/j.pragma.2013.02.010.
Tebble, H. 2009. What can interpreters learn from discourse studies. In S. Hale, U. Ozolins, and L. Stern (Eds.), *The Critical Link 5: Quality in interpreting—A shared responsibility* (pp. 201–219). John Benjamins. https://doi.org/10.1075/btl.87.16teb.
Tebble, H. 2014. A genre-based approach to teaching dialogue interpreting: The medical consultation. *The Interpreter and Translator Trainer* 8 (3): 418–436. https://doi.org/10.1080/1750399X.2014.972651.
Tiselius, E., and M. Albl-Mikasa. 2019. Introduction to the special thematic section on cognitive processes in dialogue interpreting. *Translation, Cognition and Behavior* 2 (2): 233–239. https://doi.org/10.1075/tcb.00027.tis.
Valero-Garcés, C. 2007. Doctor-patient consultations in dyadic and triadic exchanges. In F. Pöchhacker, and M. Shlesinger (Eds.), *Healthcare interpreting* (pp. 35–51). John Benjamins. https://doi.org/10.1075/bct.9.05val.
van Dijk, T.A. (Ed.). 1985. *Handbook of discourse analysis*. Academic Press.
van Dijk, T.A., and W. Kintsch. 1983. *Strategies of discourse comprehension*. Academic Press.
Wadensjö, C. 1998. *Interpreting as Interaction*. Longman.

Wadensjö, C. 2001. Approaching interpreting through discourse analysis. In D. Gile, H.V. Dam, F. Dubslaff, B. Martinsen, and A. Schjoldager (Eds.), *Getting started in interpreting research. Methodological reflections, personal accounts and advice for beginners* (pp. 185–198). John Benjamins. https://doi.org/10.1075/btl.33.12wad.

White, S.J. (2015). Closing clinical consultations. In A. Busch, and T. Spranz-Fogasy (Eds.), *Handbuch Sprache in der Medizin* (pp. 170–187). de Gruyter. https://doi.org/10.1515/9783110296174-010.

Michaela Albl-Mikasa is Professor of Interpreting Studies at the Institute of Translation and Interpreting, ZHAW Zurich University of Applied Sciences in Switzerland, where she teaches on both the BA and MA programmes. Her research and publications focus on ITELF (interpreting, translation and English as a lingua franca), the cognitive foundations of conference and community interpreting, note-taking for consecutive interpreting, the development of interpreting expertise, and medical interpreting. She was a member of the Executive Council of the International Association for Translation and Intercultural Studies (IATIS) from 2016–2021 and has been a member of the Board of the European Network of Public Service Interpreting (ENPSIT) since 2020. She is also a member of the Swiss Research Centre Barrier-free Communication and principal investigator of the interdisciplinary Sinergia project Cognitive Load in Interpreting and Translation (CLINT) funded by the Swiss National Science Foundation (SNSF). She is editor, together with Elisabet Tiselius, of the Routledge Handbook of Conference Interpreting.

Christiane Hohenstein holds a Dr. Phil. in Linguistics and a Master's Degree in Germanic Studies and Japanese Studies (both University of Hamburg), and a Certificate for Teaching in Higher Education. She is also a trainer in Continuing Education with almost 20 years of experience. She is currently a Professor for Intercultural Studies and Linguistic Diversity at Zurich University of Applied Studies, and Coordinator of a Continuing Education Program in Intercultural Studies at ZHAW's School of Applied Linguistics. Her recent research covers multilingual healthcare communication, assistive and augmentative communication, the situation of Swiss German Sign language in Higher Education, and gender sensitive and inclusive language. She has published a book with Iudicium based on her doctoral thesis on German and Japanese academic discourse, contributed papers in Journals and compilations with Benjamins, de Gruyter and Peter Lang, among others, and recently edited a book on multilingual healthcare with SMagdalène Lévy-Tödter (2020, Springer).

A Literature Review on Gender in Interpreting: Implications for Healthcare Interpreting

Carmen Acosta Vicente

1 Introduction

Public service interpreting (PSI) is a fundamental element of modern, multicultural societies, as it ensures that individuals have equal access to public services (Bancroft 2015). Considering the increased mobility in today's world, good-quality interpreting services in public service settings, such as healthcare, are an essential requirement for a participatory civil society. In addition, PSI plays a key role in the integration of migrant communities. In the case of healthcare, good-quality interpreting services also mean reduced costs for the system and better patient safety, as patients can communicate their health concerns effectively and receive the care they require at the right time (Flores 2005).

Healthcare interpreting is a complex interactional setting that typically involves three participants (with different roles, expectations, and social identities) in an act of communication. One of the most salient of such social identities is gender, as we use it as a basic parameter to categorise the people we interact with in order to make sense of the situations we take part in (Germon 2009). For instance, there is a general understanding that gender is a relevant factor in doctor-patient interaction (Hall et al. 1994; Cousin et al. 2013; Chakraverty et al. 2020, among others). However, little attention has been paid to gender in interpreter-mediated healthcare encounters, and the literature on gender in interpreting remains scarce (Baer and Missardier-Kenney 2015).

There are many approaches to and perspectives on the concept of *gender* and its meaning—for instance, we can talk about social gender or gender identity; we can understand gender as a binary system or as one that comprises multiple gender identities; or we can refer to gender as a category independent from sex or as one

C. Acosta Vicente (✉)
University of Helsinki, Helsinki, Finland
e-mail: carmen.acostavicente@helsinki.fi

R. Lázaro Gutiérrez and C. Álvaro Aranda (eds.), *New Trends in Healthcare Interpreting Studies*, New Frontiers in Translation Studies,
https://doi.org/10.1007/978-981-99-2961-0_3

that is interconnected with it (Butler 1988; 2004; Harrison 2006; Pavlidou 2011). This diversity shows the complexity of gender and may present methodological challenges. However, it also provides a rich range of possibilities for the study of gender in healthcare interpreting.

In this chapter, I present a literature review on gender in interpreting through a qualitative meta-synthesis. This literature review aims to provide a clear picture of the state of research on the topic of gender in interpreting and identify the research areas that healthcare interpreting studies may explore to acquire a better understanding of the topic in that context. In view of the variety of angles that can be taken in the study of gender, this literature review does not focus on a single understanding or definition of *gender*, but on how *gender* (however it is understood) is problematised in the literature regarding interpreting. Thus, this chapter analyses how the literature has explored and problematised gender-related issues in interpreting by looking at academic publications dealing with gender from interpreting studies and adjacent disciplines.

In Sect. 2, I offer a brief overview of gender issues in healthcare interaction. In Sects. 3–6, I present the focus of this chapter: a literature review on gender in interpreting, which covers a selection of relevant monographs and journals in interpreting studies and adjacent disciplines and draws out the implications they have for healthcare interpreting. Section 3 provides information on the methods and data used for the literature review. In Sect. 4, the studies are thematically categorised and analysed. This is followed by a discussion of the findings of the literature review and their implications for healthcare interpreting in Sect. 5. Section 6 presents the conclusions of the chapter, which provide a summary of the main themes identified in the literature and propose suggestions for further research on gender in healthcare interpreting.

2 Gender in Healthcare Interaction

Institutional interaction in healthcare settings has received significant attention since the 1960s, with many contributions made to the understanding of social structures, institutional language use, and the dyadic nature of doctor-patient communication, among other areas (Heritage and Maynard 2011). The relationship between healthcare professionals (HCPs) and their patients is crucial to patients' state of health and may determine their attitude towards the treatment they are receiving and towards medicine overall (ibid.). Therefore, the findings of communication-oriented studies in healthcare can provide insights into processes that have the potential to change people's lives.

Conversation analysis has shown that institutional talk and common conversation are fairly similar types of verbal interaction. For instance, doctors and patients do not abandon usual interactional conventions when they meet in a healthcare context. Rather, they adapt to the new setting according to their understanding of what is and what is not appropriate for the context (ibid.). Thus, it can also be inferred that doctors' and patients' other social identities do not disappear in medical contexts: they are still present in their roles as *doctor* and *patient*. The same applies to those performing the interpreter's role (Angelelli 2001), which is an important aspect to consider when exploring the issue of gender in interpreter-mediated interaction.

The impact that gender may have on the way doctor-patient interaction is constructed has been explored from different perspectives. For instance, Hall et al. (1994) and Cousin et al. (2013) analysed gender differences in communicative outcomes. Their findings suggest that a power struggle may arise between male patients and female doctors. Furthermore, studies have found that gender influences how much patients trust their practitioner and how comfortable they feel discussing certain topics. This is particularly significant in the case of migrant communities due to cultural differences in what is considered appropriate gendered behaviour. Some outcomes of gender mismatches between patients and HCPs include patients withholding information because they feel ashamed of disclosing it to someone of a different gender to them, or patients refusing treatment altogether (Roussos et al. 2010; Chakraverty et al. 2020).

While numerous studies on healthcare interaction have focused on a dyadic model of communication, there is also a smaller—but growing—number of studies that focus on the very particular interaction that occurs when an interpreter joins the usually dyadic communication between HCPs and patients (see, for instance, Valero Garcés 2005 and Levinger 2020). According to Wadensjö (1998), interpreter-mediated interaction is usually seen as a deviation from normality and a communication burden instead of simply as a different communication model combining dyadic and triadic communication. Focusing on the latter, Wadensjö argues that the interpreter is an inherent participant in the interaction, acting both as a translator and a mediator. This understanding shows a more realistic representation of the interpreter's role in healthcare settings. Angelelli's (2004) findings regarding interpreters' perception of their role support this view. Her work shows that medical interpreters (representing community interpreting as a whole in her monograph) consider themselves significantly more visible in interactions than conference and court interpreters do. They see themselves not as linguistic conduits but as participants in the interaction who may, for instance, experience alignment with the parties, or contribute to the development of trust between the parties (Angelelli 2001). If the interpreter's visibility makes it possible for the interpreter's social background to become relevant in the interaction (ibid.) and if interpreters' own perceptions signal that medical encounters make them particularly visible, is it not fair to assume that gender plays a role worth exploring in this area?

3 Methods and Data

I conducted a meta-synthesis by analysing the way in which the literature in interpreting has dealt with gender-related issues. The corpus included chapters from *The Critical Link* conference proceedings (1–6) and articles from translation and interpreting (T&I) journals (*Interpreting: International Journal of Research and Practice in Interpreting, The International Journal of Translation and Interpreting Research, Translation and Interpreting Studies, Target: International Journal of Translation Studies, The International Journal of Interpreter Education, Perspectives: Studies in Translation Theory and Practice, The Journal of Interpretation v.19–29*). These sources were selected because they provide a large number of studies for the search and are reliable in terms of the quality of publications. The terms selected for the search were *gender* and *sex*. *Sex* was included in the term search because *gender* and *sex* are sometimes used interchangeably. The results of the term search are presented in Table 1.

The resources used were available online, and I used the journals' online search tools to perform the term search. I wanted to select studies in which *gender* had significance. Hence, I decided to limit my search to journal articles where the terms appeared in the abstract, the title, or the subject terms, which I did by using the advanced search tools in the online versions of the journals.

However, this method was not suitable for *The Critical Link* conference proceedings, as they are compiled in monograph format and the search tool available in the electronic version does not allow for refined search parameters. In this case, I did a manual search of the chapters contained in each one of the conference proceedings (1–6) and selected those that contained the abovementioned terms in any part of the text. I went through each chapter and removed those in which the terms were only mentioned in the bibliography or did not relate to interpreting, the interpreter, or any of the participants in the interpreter-mediated encounter. Since the selection method was different to the one used for the journals, the data from the conference proceedings is presented in a separate row in Table 1.

The first search provided few results, indicating that this research topic has not yet been thoroughly explored in interpreting studies, and even less so in healthcare interpreting (only three of the articles in the T&I journals and conference proceedings referred to healthcare). Since the data obtained was considered too limited to provide a solid perspective on this topic, an additional search was conducted by looking at sources and materials from adjacent fields within the scope of the topic of the literature review, such as healthcare and gender studies. I found these articles by using general search methods, namely *Google Scholar*, the *Helka* online database of the University of Helsinki libraries, and by searching through the reference section of previously found articles dealing with gender in interpreting. The findings from these sources are presented in a separate row in Table 1.

It is worth mentioning that the number of articles including the term *gender* in the interpreting journals is higher than that shown in Table 1. Those articles, which have not been included in the corpus, mention *gender* only as a variable to categorise

Table 1 Number of articles resulting from the term search for *gender* and *sex* categorised by the source of the materials

T&I Journals	N. of articles on *gender*	N. of articles on *sex*	CL Conference Proceedings	N. of articles on *gender*	N. of articles on *sex*	Other sources	N. of articles/ monographs
Interpreting: international journal of research and practice in interpreting	2	0	CL1 (1995)	0	0	Journals in other fields (gender studies, healthcare, linguistics)	10
The international journal of translation and interpreting research	3	0	CL2 (1998)	0	0	Monographs	2
The journal of interpretation	2	0	CL3 (2001)	3	0	Conference papers	1
Translation and interpreting studies	1	0	CL4 (2004)	0	1		
Target: international journal of translation studies	1	0	CL5 (2009)	1	2		
Perspectives: studies in translation theory and practice	6	0	CL6 (2013)	2	0		
International journal of interpreter education	1	0					
Total	16	0		6	3		13

participants during the data collection or list it among other variables that might have influenced the findings, but they do not problematise gender in any way.

As a final remark on the methodology, this review is limited by the materials available in the search engines and databases used and by the language of the materials (all the articles and chapters included in this review are in English, except for one in Spanish). Other suitable materials may be available in other languages or fields.

4 Analysis

In this section, the search results are categorised thematically and analysed. The analysis includes articles from all interpreting settings due to the limited results obtained on gender in healthcare interpreting alone. I saw this as an indicator that in order to explore the role of gender in healthcare interpreting, we must first examine the findings of the overall literature on interpreting. Before proceeding with the thematic analysis, two main conclusions can be already drawn from the results of Table 1.

First, research on the topic of gender in interpreting studies is limited (16 articles in T&I studies journals, 9 chapters in *The Critical Link* conference proceedings, and 13 articles in other sources). Even though there is a clear gap in research concerning the interpreter's social identities and their significance to their professional practice, issues connected with gender and the interpreter's social identities have been extensively researched. For instance, a quick search of the term *role* in the journal *Interpreting* yielded 58 results, and there were 10 chapters dealing with the interpreter's agency in the fourth volume of *The Critical Link* conference proceedings alone. This suggests that there is a solid background for conducting research on gender in interpreting, and that this context is favourable for research in this area to grow. Furthermore, the literature on interpreting studies often mentions *gender* or uses it to categorise participants (e.g. Schwenke 2012; Yenkimaleki and van Heuven 2018), but questions regarding how and to what extent the participants' gender affects the findings they present or why it may be relevant remain unanswered. In other words, there appears to be a general understanding that these matters influence interpreting in some way, but gender as such is not problematised.

Second, there is an overwhelming preference for the term *gender* over *sex* in the interpreting literature. In fact, not a single instance of the term *sex* could be found in the interpreting journals, and the three instances identified in the conference proceedings only used the term *sex* as a variable to classify the participants but presented no further analysis on it.

The strategy to narrow down the journal articles to those including the search terms in the title, abstract, or subject terms was useful for finding articles dealing with gender. However, there were a few articles in which the term *gender* did appear in one of those sections, but where the article did not cover matters related to gender. I did not categorise those articles by theme (see Table 2, value X).

4.1 Interpreting and Gender: Themes

To analyse the data, I divided the articles into four categories based on their orientation to gender: studies analysing gender differences based on the interpreter's gender (I); studies focusing on the gendered behaviours and perceptions of interpreters (II); studies focusing on the interpreter's rendition of gendered language or gendered

Table 2 Number of articles and chapters per theme

Sources	I	II	III	IV	X (Topic not covered)
T&I journals	7	3	1	2	3
CL	1	0	0	3	5
Other sources	3	1	2	7	0
Total number	11	4	3	12	8

discourse (III); and studies focusing on various aspects related to gender dynamics between the participants in interpreter-mediated encounters (IV). As shown in Table 2, themes I and IV are the best represented in the literature.

4.1.1 Gender Differences (I)

The first category refers to the literature that compares men and women in their role as interpreters. The literature has explored these differences through various lenses, namely role and status, interpreter training, and gender differences in language use.

In terms of the interpreter's role, Angelelli was, to my knowledge, one of the first scholars to look at gender in relation to the interpreter's perception of their role. She examined interpreters' perceptions against their social background using data obtained through a survey of court, conference, and medical interpreters in Canada, the United States, and Mexico. The results of the paper published in the third volume of *The Critical Link* conference proceedings (Angelelli 2001) indicated that there were gender differences in the way interpreters perceived their role; however, the paper did not specify the nature of those differences. In contrast, the findings presented in Angelelli's monograph on the same topic (2004) showed no significant gender differences in the interpreters' perception of their role. Using a global survey, Gentile (2018) analysed gender differences in conference interpreters' perceptions of the status, prestige, and social value of their profession. Similarly to Angelelli's findings, the results showed no significant gender differences in terms of self-perception. However, the female participants believed that laypeople considered their profession to have a significantly lower status, prestige, and social value compared with the perceptions of their male counterparts. Gentile pointed out that this may impact interpreters' self-esteem and confidence at work.

Other studies have analysed gender differences in the context of difficulties encountered by interpreters in training. Valero Garcés and Socarrás-Estrada (2012) included gender as a variable in their study on assessment and evaluation in PSI training labs at the University of Alcalá (Madrid, Spain) by measuring the interpreting skills of 137 students before and after receiving PSI training. Their analysis on the correlation between accuracy, speed response, and stress tolerance mentions that women outperformed men overall, but men showed better stress tolerance.

However, these results are not further explored or problematized. Pan and Xiu Yan (2012) conducted a study with 77 interpreting students in China, which reviewed the students' perceptions of their learning patterns and correlated them with their socio-biographical background. Concerning gender, the results indicated that, based on their own perceptions, male students had more linguistic and fluency problems. These results are compatible with the findings of studies on gender differences in language learning. Nonetheless, the authors stated that their findings provided no evidence that women outperformed men in the interpreting training process, as there is more to interpreting than its linguistic aspects. They also highlighted that more studies on gender differences in interpreting strategies and output are necessary to compare the findings and examine whether there are clear gender patterns that should be considered during interpreting training.

Several studies have focused on gender differences in interpreting output—in other words, on whether men and women interpret differently. One of those is Nakane's (2008) study, which investigated gender and politeness in Japanese-English police interpreting in Australia. Nakane found that women used significantly more honorifics than men when interpreting into Japanese. However, the author pointed out that, in Japanese, honorifics are not only used to perform femininity; they may also signal status, level of education, and sophistication. Therefore, the connection between the use of honorifics and traditional perceptions of "women's language" should not be taken for granted but should be further problematised.

The literature on conference interpreting has shown a greater interest in differences in language use than has the literature on PSI. This can be seen in the work of Magnifico and Defrancq (2016, 2017, 2019, 2020), who examined gender differences in conference interpreting in the European Parliament using the EPICG (European Parliament Interpreting Corpus Ghent) corpus. For their analysis, the authors selected 39 speeches in French and 39 interpretations in Dutch and English. Their study on impoliteness (Magnifico and Defrancq 2016) looked at how interpreters handled face-threatening acts (FTAs) and revealed that male interpreters were more prone to using mitigation as a strategy to deal with impoliteness, contrary to the common belief that women are more inclined to use softening strategies. As a potential explanation for female interpreters' lower use of mitigation, the authors suggested that they may place a higher value on professional norms. These results are contradicted by Bartłomiejczyk's (2020) later study on impoliteness in Polish interpretations of UKIP's Eurosceptic discourse at the European Parliament, which did not find significant gender differences in the interpreters' mitigation strategies.

Magnifico and Defrancq's (2019) findings on the use of self-repairs showed that women use self-repairs more frequently. Again, the authors associated this phenomenon with a difference in interpreters' adherence to norms under the premise that female interpreters tend to seek the most precise terms in their output. Yet, when it comes to the use of editing terms, the study found no clear gender differences, and disparate results were acquired depending on the language pair. Their study on interpreters' use of hedges (Magnifico and Defrancq 2017) also showed no significant gender differences. In their article on connective markers, Magnifico and Defrancq (2020) specifically looked at the connection between gender differences and adherence to professional norms that had been previously identified. As was the case regarding the use of hedges, they did not find any connection between the interpreters' gender and their rendition of connective markers; instead, they found that the speed of the speech delivery influences the rendition of connective markers. As a whole, these findings present a complex picture of the topic and do not make it possible to identify a clear pattern regarding gender differences in the interpreters' output in conference interpreting.

Hu and Meng (2018) also contributed to this area with their study on gender differences in the linguistic choices made by interpreters in Chinese-English press conferences. They analysed data from the Chinese-English conference interpreting corpus 3.0 developed by the Centre for Translation and Intercultural Studies at Shanghai Jiao Tong University. The authors ascribed the differences identified to existing gender roles in China, where there is a significant gender-related power imbalance. They argued, similarly to Magnifico and Defrancq, that female interpreters' higher inclination towards accuracy is due to their stronger adherence to norms and that male interpreters' tendency to provide more creative outputs results from their greater freedom to express themselves.

4.1.2 The Interpreter's Gender: Behaviours and Perceptions (II)

This theme refers to the interpreter's gender and relates to both the interpreter's behaviour and the perception others might have of it. On this theme, the literature on conference interpreting and PSI has focused on two different areas.

The literature on conference interpreting has explored the gendered perceptions broader audiences have of interpreters. Ellcessor (2015) analysed media responses to Lydia Callis and Holly Maniatty, two American Sign Language (ASL) interpreters who have covered mainstream events with high visibility among hearing audiences. In her analysis, Ellcessor reported that the public's problematic response to the interpreters—which involved ridiculing and mocking—is linked to a gendered spectacularisation of ASL interpreting. Taking a similar focus on the way women are perceived in their role as interpreters, Cho (2017) undertook a qualitative survey study of Korean-English interpreting graduates. The survey obtained 27 responses, of which 26 came from female respondents. In her article, she discussed the growing focus in South Korea on the personal aesthetics of female interpreters. The results of her study showed that female interpreters perform aesthetic labour in addition to language work to meet the requirements of a competitive and oversaturated language market. These studies present evidence that gendered perceptions of interpreters have an impact on their profession and that women are subjected to sexism in their work as interpreters.

The literature on PSI has explored gender issues among migrant women who become interpreters in their host country. Iliescu Gheorghiu (2012) interviewed eight female Romanian ad hoc interpreters who assisted family members in accessing healthcare in Spain. She found that the cultural differences linked to medical experiences in the Romanian and Spanish healthcare systems affected the way the interpreters and patients perceived bodily issues in medical contexts. Participants stated that they felt more at ease participating in medical encounters in Spain due to the smaller power asymmetry between the parties. They also stated that they felt more comfortable disclosing and discussing bodily matters in the Spanish system, and they did not experience the feeling of inferiority to the degree they did in Romanian healthcare contexts.

Lee et al. (2016) conducted a qualitative study on the community interpreting services provided by Multicultural Family Support Centres to help migrant women integrate into South Korean society. They interviewed 23 interpreters –who were also migrant women– and 10 of their supervisors. Regarding the interpreters' role and status, the study revealed that the interpreters performed tasks that far exceeded what would be considered strictly interpreting. In addition, the findings indicated that the interpreters often became fundamental support for the migrant women they assisted while also facing stigma and discrimination due to their own status as migrants. Furthermore, they were not considered professional interpreters and, even though they achieved a high status in their communities, their social status in South Korean society remained rather low, which is a common trend in work performed by women (Holbrook 1991; Cortina 2006).

4.1.3 Rendition of Gendered Language and Discourse (III)

This category refers to the interpreter's management of gendered language or gendered discourse. One of the specific topics explored is the interpretation of gendered language and grammatical gender. Both Quinto-Pozos et al. (2015) and McDermid et al. (2021) analysed this issue through observing the decisions made by interpreters working with ASL (which lacks gender-markedness in pronouns) and English and Spanish (where pronouns can be gender-marked). The findings of these studies identified strategies that interpreters implement to deal with the lack of gender markers and revealed that many interpreters made assumptions based on stereotypes or, in the case of Spanish, used masculine forms by default. They also identified strategies used to maintain the gender-neutral nature of the source, the most common ones being the use of the pronoun *they* and the use of vague noun phrase agents to avoid specifying gender. These studies show how language use may reveal the interpreter's gender-related beliefs when dealing with gendered or gender-neutral language.

Maryns (2013) analysed interactional data to examine the (re)performance of gendered discourse in an interpreter-mediated asylum interview. The article explored how the asylum-seeker's identity was co-constructed and reperformed by the asylum officer and, most saliently, by the interpreter. The analysis shows how the interpreter (female) reperformed the narration of episodes of sexual violence experienced by the asylum-seeker (male) with significantly different connotations, which might be associated with the interpreter feeling uncomfortable with the topic or the words used by the asylum-seeker. The author notes that (re)performance is present in the encounter in several ways (gender performance, entextualisation of the asylum-seeker´s testimony, and translation itself), which highlights the complexity behind the rendition of gendered discourse. Thus, she proposes that the management of gender-based claims is oriented toward individual cognition instead of relying on homogeneous guidelines that are not always beneficial considering the heterogeneous nature of these encounters.

4.1.4 Gender Dynamics in Interpreter-Mediated Interaction (IV)

The literature has looked at gender dynamics between participants and its impact on communication in interpreter-mediated interaction from a variety of angles. MacDougall's (2012) article on gendered discourse in ASL interpreting studies indicated the potential of gender research in this area. She reviewed studies principally dealing with politeness and credibility in ASL, and her work brings out two main themes regarding the issue of gender in ASL interpreting. The first one relates to power dominance expressed through language, taking into consideration the fact that the ASL interpreting field is mostly composed of white women. The second theme addresses the need to include gender issues in training curricula to improve interpreters' sensitivity to gender dynamics and how their own social identities have an impact on their profession.

In addition, some studies have addressed the relationship between gender and culture in interpreting. Crezee (2001) conducted a small pilot survey for healthcare interpreters in New Zealand to explore issues related to cultural barriers in interpreter-mediated communication. The issue of gender was mentioned by 2% of the respondents. Even though the percentage was small, their responses suggested that cultural background may create gender issues when the interpreter's gender does not match the patient's. Osman and Angelelli (2011) also analysed the cultural and religious perceptions of gender roles in interpreter-mediated interaction in the context of the court case of Sheikh Omar Abdel-Rahman. In particular, they looked at transcriptions of the subsequent interviews he had with his lawyer (a woman) and his interpreter (a man). Their interactional analysis showed that the interpreter was the most active participant in the interaction and created an Arabic-centred discourse that established culturally appropriate gendered behaviours while either making substantial additions to the lawyer's utterances, including cultural conventions, or avoiding rendering the lawyer's interventions. In this way, the female lawyer became a passive interlocutor in a situation where she would have been expected to have a crucial role.

Issues related to interpreting in cases of gender-based violence have also been studied. Oda and Joyette (2001) examined gender in their efforts to design a screening tool for interpreter training programmes to work with perpetrators of domestic abuse. Their assessment provided no concrete evidence that the interpreter's gender would be either beneficial or detrimental to communication. However, the study by Lehti et al. (2021) found that women were preferred as interpreters in cases of gender-based violence in order to create a more comfortable and trusting environment for the victim in situations concerning women's psychological health issues. Their data, collected in six EU countries, was based on the analysis of journal entries written by service providers working with refugee women who had suffered gender-based violence. Their findings suggested that clients preferred female doctors and interpreters, and that interpreters played a fundamental role in fostering or hindering the development of trust between the service providers and the service seekers. Within the context of the European pilot project *Speak Out for Support* (SOS-VICS), Valero Garcés et al. (2015) provided a comprehensive description of the protocol followed within the Spanish healthcare system in cases of gender-based violence and discussed deontological aspects of the interpreter's role. The authors argued that interpreters play a fundamental role in guaranteeing the victims' rights, that interpreters should be part of the teams handling the cases, and that they should be prepared to handle the emotional toll of the work setting. Within the Australian context, Norma and García-Caro (2016) argued for the need for specialised interpreting training on issues related to gender-based violence. They examined official reports from governmental and non-governmental organisations as well as the findings from academic literature related to gender issues concerning interpreting in cases of gender-violence. In their analysis, they linked the lack of this type of specialised interpreting training to a narrow understanding of professional standards related to the interpreter's impartiality. Even though the focus of these studies varies, all of them highlight the importance of the interpreter's sensitivity and competence in cases of gender-based violence, which calls for specific gender-related training.

The importance of the gender of the participants in interpreter-mediated healthcare encounters has also been explored in healthcare literature, from guidelines on how to work with interpreters (Hadziabdic and Hjelm 2013) –which recommend matching the interpreter's gender to the patient's when discussing sensitive issues– to the role gender plays in how comfortable the patient feels, to doctor and patient satisfaction with communication outcomes (Roussos et al. 2010; Mengesha et al. 2018; Chakraverty et al. 2020). The connection between patient and doctor satisfaction and gender echoes the findings of Stone's (2013) study, which included a small survey of British sign-language interpreters. Gender was signalled as a relevant factor for client satisfaction, but this was not further problematised. Thus, more data would be required to establish the nature of the link between the two.

In any case, gender seems to play an important role in healthcare interpreting. This was stated by Roussos et al. (2010) when explaining their motivation to look at gender regarding interpreter-mediated communication in healthcare in the United States: "Given no prior evidence to suspect that gender would play a role in interpreting, this qualitative study was not planned to identify the role of gender. To our surprise, the topic of gender was unavoidable" (Roussos et al. 2010: 220). Their study consisted of focus groups with monolingual HCPs, male Latino patients, and bilingual staff working as interpreters, which indicated that gender is not a relevant factor for impartiality, cultural awareness, respect, or professionalism. However, the findings showed that gender visibility in interaction caused different reactions from participants and recommended that interpreters have the same gender as the patient when appropriate and that gender issues be included in interpreter training programmes. In addition,

Mengesha et al. (2018) conducted 21 interviews with HCPs in Australia regarding the participation of interpreters in sexual and reproductive health discussions with migrant women. Their findings showed that healthcare providers were reluctant to use male interpreters because that could prevent the patients from discussing sensitive topics or disclosing whether they are being subjected to violence. They also indicated that there are not enough female interpreters to cover the linguistic needs of emerging migrant communities. Accordingly, they called for the recruitment and training of more female interpreters from non-English speaking backgrounds. Lastly, Chakraverty et al. (2020) conducted focus groups with HCPs in Germany that examined HCPs' perceptions of gender-specific aspects of health literacy when working with migrant communities. The results revealed that HCPs believed it necessary to work with interpreters who act as cultural mediators to navigate gender issues.

5 Discussion

The fact that gender has not received much attention in the literature on healthcare interpreting to date might not come as a surprise. As we saw in the previous section, this is not because gender is irrelevant to the field, but because interpreting as an area of study is broad, complex, and multidisciplinary, and there are still many topics within healthcare interpreting that remain unexplored. Nonetheless, in this chapter, we have seen that steps have already been taken with regard to the study of gender in interpreting. In this section, I will discuss how the existing literature shines some light on the role of gender in healthcare interpreting. Before that, it is important to present four observations regarding the overall characteristics of the literature included in this review.

First, the gender issues explored to date vary greatly and include a wide range of topics within the interpreting field, such as interpreting training, the interpreter's role and status, and interpreters' language use. However, the limited number of studies in each area implies that the findings may provide only a small glimpse of the issue in question. For instance, the findings by Pan and Xiu Yan (2012) indicated that the male interpreting students in their sample had more linguistic and fluency problems during training; however, these findings by themselves do not provide conclusive evidence that male interpreting students struggle more than their female counterparts during training.

Second, most of the studies reviewed in this chapter are qualitative studies focusing on a specific moment in time, place, and dataset. In other words, the types of studies undertaken to date do not allow for any generalisations to be made or clear conclusions to be drawn. I anticipated this before undertaking the review, as gender is a relatively new topic in interpreting studies, and therefore foresaw that research on gender would be of an exploratory nature.

Third, only 13 of the 38 sources identified through the term search presented a clear definition of *gender*. Most sources used *gender* as if there was a general understanding of what it is and provided no information on its meaning. Furthermore, the predominant trend is to refer to a binary categorisation of gender (men/women), which shows a narrow perspective on gender issues. As noted in the introduction, there are many approaches to gender. In order to acquire solid knowledge on gender in interpreting and, specifically, in healthcare interpreting, it is important to first establish what we are referring to and acknowledge that gender as a category goes beyond the binary (Butler 2004).

Fourth, the data presented in the studies mostly consisted of surveys, interviews, or focus groups. With a few exceptions (Nakane 2008; Osman and Angelelli 2011; Maryns 2013), there is little empirical interactional evidence taken directly from interpreter-mediated encounters. Thus, interactional analysis of gender in interpreter-mediated communication is very limited. Conducting more research along these lines is necessary in order to acquire a comprehensive understanding of the role played by gender in interpreting. Otherwise, our knowledge of this research area will be limited to beliefs and perceptions of gender.

These observations do not detract from the value of the studies. Each one of them has offered an initial answer to some of the many questions arising from the issue of gender in interpreting, and they provide a basis for future research.

In terms of healthcare interpreting, this chapter has shown that medical interpreters rank high in terms of their visibility in the communication event (Angelelli 2001), and that gender in itself plays an important role in healthcare settings due to the kinds of issues disclosed in such contexts –e.g. regarding sexual and reproductive health. Therefore, it is fair to assume that healthcare interpreting provides favourable conditions for conducting gender research. However, only eight of the articles reviewed related to healthcare interpreting, and four of them came from the healthcare field. Consequently, the findings have their own limitations for interpreting studies, since they show a different understanding of interpreting and the interpreter's role. Nonetheless, these results, as well as the findings from other interpreting settings, have significant implications for healthcare interpreting.

The results indicate that gender is relevant in healthcare interpreting. There is reason to believe that the interpreter's gender has an impact on how comfortable the patient feels and on establishing trust between the parties. The connection between gender and trust in community interpreting is implicit in the work of Lee et al. (2016) and explicit in the work of Lehti et al. (2021). This has direct implications for healthcare interpreting, as interpreters have an important role in the development of trust between healthcare providers and their patients (Nicodemus et al. 2020). In addition, the findings of Roussos et al. (2010), Mengesha et al. (2018), and Chakraverty et al. (2020) highlight the interpreter's visibility in healthcare encounters and indicate that gender is a factor to consider in interpreter-mediated interaction to ensure patients feel comfortable disclosing information, especially when dealing with taboos rooted in cultural perceptions of gender issues. However, it is worth noting that healthcare studies in this area do not include empirical interactional data of interpreter-mediated encounters, so the interactional complexity of interpreter-mediated communication and the impact of gender in such interaction remain unanalysed. Therefore, more research coming from the interpreting field is necessary.

Furthermore, these issues are linked to the connection between gender and culture (Crezee 2001; Osman and Angelelli 2011). Given the sensitivity of the topics discussed in healthcare settings, exploring how cultural and ideological perceptions of gender held by medical interpreters, HCPs, and patients affect the interactional dynamics in healthcare interactions may yield interesting results.

Institutional differences also appear to be relevant from a gender perspective. Iliescu Gheorghiu's (2012) study indicates that power imbalances related to gender differ depending on the cultural and institutional healthcare context, and those power dynamics impose certain behavioural rules. This could potentially affect the interpreter's behaviour, for example, when it comes to turn-taking, the level of formality expected in the interaction, or the kinds of topics that are deemed appropriate to discuss in a medical context. Thus, this is worth considering when providing training for medical interpreters. Likewise, following the work of Oda and Joyette (2001), Valero Garcés, et al. (2015), and Norma and García-Caro (2016), attention should be paid to gender issues and gender-based violence in healthcare interpreting training programmes, as these are highly relevant for healthcare interpreting and require specific knowledge, awareness, and sensitivity.

The findings regarding the interpreter's rendition of gendered language and discourse (Maryns 2013; Quinto-Pozos et al. 2015; McDermid et al. 2021) have important implications for healthcare interpreting in terms of the interpreter's sensitivity towards such matters. In fact, the interpreter's pronoun choice and use of gender-marked words can be crucial in healthcare interaction, for instance, during medical encounters with transgender patients. However, the results of the interpreting literature on gender differences in language use provide a more heterogeneous picture. There is potential to conduct similar studies to Nakane's (2008) in the context of healthcare interpreting to identify possible gender differences in the way interpreters manage the power dynamics of healthcare interaction when dealing with politeness and FTAs. However, in terms of the phenomena explored by Magnifico and Defrancq (2016, 2017, 2019, 2020), Hu and Meng (2018), and Bartłomiejczyk (2020), it is difficult to determine if the same differences would be identified, or if they would even be amplified in the context of healthcare interpreting, where the interpreter is more visible. Nonetheless, following the findings of Magnifico and Defrancq (2016, 2017, 2019, 2020) and Hu and Meng (2018), it would be interesting to analyse potential gender differences in the adherence to professional norms in healthcare interpreting –for instance, whether women have a stronger focus on remaining neutral in their role as interpreters, as neutrality is required by many healthcare interpreting guidelines.

Lastly, as in any other human activity, gender roles, perceptions, and expectations have an impact on interpreting (Osman and Angelelli 2011; MacDougall 2012; Maryns 2013; Ellcessor 2015; Cho 2017; Gentile, 2018; Hu and Meng 2018) and on the dynamics of the participants in interaction in healthcare settings (Hall et al. 1994; Cousin et al. 2013). For instance, when applied to healthcare interpreting, the studies by Ellcessor (2015) and Cho (2017) raise the question of how healthcare providers' and patients' gender beliefs may affect their perception of the interpreter and their attitudes towards them, for example, in terms of the trust and credibility they grant them. How these issues materialise in healthcare interpreting and the outcomes they might produce are crucial areas to explore.

6 Conclusions

This chapter has provided a review of the literature on gender in interpreting and explored its implications for healthcare interpreting. The review covered a total of 30 articles taken from T&I journals, *The Critical Link* conference proceedings (1–6), and additional material from adjacent fields. The articles and chapters were divided into four categories, and sub-themes were identified.

The literature review showed that most of the studies conducted to date are qualitative, and the predominant data sources were surveys, interviews, and focus groups. More research (both qualitative and quantitative) and interactional data from interpreter-mediated communication are needed to acquire a broader perspective on the issue and for this research area to develop. Most of the studies reviewed deal with *gender* as a social category and refer to the gender of the interpreter or the client, but the review also includes studies dealing with how interpreters render gendered language, for instance. Regardless of their focus, future studies would benefit from including clear definitions of *gender* as their subject of study instead of relying on an intuitive understanding of *gender*.

The findings analysed in this chapter do not allow generalisations due to the limited research available. However, they present conjectures that call for further research and that could be applied to and explored in healthcare interpreting. The most significant ones are as follows:

- Interpreters perceive their role and professional status similarly regardless of their gender, even though perceptions of interpreters may differ socially and culturally based on gender.
- Sexism has an impact on interpreting and different perceptions of gender beliefs, roles, and expectations may materialise in interpreter-mediated interaction.
- There are gender differences in the use of linguistic features that might be linked to a higher adherence to professional norms by female interpreters, but findings in this regard are heterogeneous and sometimes contradictory.
- The interpreter's own gender assumptions and beliefs can affect their decisions when interpreting gendered language or discourse.
- Gender-related issues are closely related to cultural and institutional conventions.
- Gender-related education in interpreter training curricula is necessary to improve awareness of gender issues, especially when dealing with sensitive matters, such as sexual and reproductive health or gender-based violence.
- The interpreter's gender is relevant to how comfortable patients feel, the development of trust, and doctor and patient satisfaction with communication outcomes in healthcare interpreting.

In brief, this literature review has shown that there is limited research on gender in interpreting studies and even less so in healthcare interpreting. However, it has also shown the great potential this research area has. The comprehensive development of gender in healthcare interpreting as a research area would not only improve our understanding of the matter but would also enhance the quality of the services provided and prevent problematic situations for all parties involved.

References

Angelelli, Claudia. 2001. The interpersonal role of the interpreter in cross-cultural communication: A survey of conference, court and medical interpreters in the US, Canada and Mexico. In *The Critical Link 3: Interpreters in the Community. Selected Papers from the Third International Conference on Interpreting in Legal, Health and Social Service Settings, Montréal, Quebec, Canada 22–26 May 2001*, eds. Louise Brunette, Georges L. Bastin, Isabelle Hemlin and Heather Clark, 15–6. Amsterdam: John Benjamins.

Angelelli, Claudia, 2004. *Revisiting the interpreter's role: A study of conference, court, and medical interpreters in Canada, Mexico, and the United States*. Philadelphia: John Benjamins.

Baer, Brian James, and Françoise Massardier-Kenney. 2015. Gender and sexuality. In *Researching Translation and Interpreting*, eds. Claudia V. Angelelli and Brian James Baer, 83–96. London: Routledge

Bancroft, Marjory A. 2015. Community interpreting: A profession rooted in social justice. In *The Routledge Handbook of Interpreting*, ed. Holly Mikkelson and Renée Jourdenais, 217–235. Oxford: Routledge.

Bartłomiejczyk, Magdalena. 2020. Parliamentary impoliteness and the interpreter's gender. *Pragmatics* 30 (4): 459–484. https://doi.org/10.1075/prag.18064.bar.

Butler, Judith. 1988. Performative acts and gender constitution: An essay in phenomenology and feminist theory. *Theater Journal* 40 (4): 519–531.

Butler, Judith. 2004. *Undoing Gender*. New York: Routledge.

Chakraverty, Digo, Annika Baumeister, Angela Aldin, Tina Jakob, Ümran Sema Seven, Christiane Woopen, Nicole Skoetz, and Elke Kalbe. 2020. Gender-specific aspects of health literacy: Perceptions of interactions with migrants among health care providers in Germany. *International Journal of Environmental and Public Health* 17 (7). https://doi.org/10.3390/ijerph17072189.

Cho, Jinhyun. 2017. Why do interpreters need to be beautiful? Aesthetic labour of language workers. *Gender and Language* 11 (4): 482–506. https://doi.org/10.1558/genl.31618.

Cortina, Regina. 2006. Women teachers in Mexico: Asymmetries of power in public education. In *Women and Teaching: Global Perspectives on the Feminization of a Profession*, eds. Regina Cortina and Sonsoles San Román, 107–128. New York: Palgrave Macmillan.

Cousin, Gaetan, Marianne Schmid Mast, and Nicole Jaunin-Stalder. 2013. When physician-expressed uncertainty leads to patient dissatisfaction: A gender study. *Medical Education* 47: 923–931. https://doi.org/10.1111/medu.12237.

Crezee, Ineke. 2001. Health interpreting: The cultural divide. In *The Critical Link 3: Interpreters in the Community. Selected Papers from the Third International Conference on Interpreting in Legal, Health and Social Service Settings, Montréal, Québec, Canada 22–26 May 2001*, eds. Louise Brunette, Georges L. Bastin, Isabelle Hemlin and Heather Clark, 249–259. Amsterdam: John Benjamins.

Ellcessor, Elizabeth. 2015. Is there a sign for that? Media, American Sign Language interpretation, and the paradox of visibility. *Perspectives* 23 (4): 586–598. https://doi.org/10.1080/0907676X.2015.1056814.

Flores, Glenn. 2005. The impact of medical interpreter services on the quality of health care: A systematic review. *Medical Care Research and Review* 62 (3): 255–299. https://doi.org/10.1177/1077558705275416.

Gentile, Paola. 2018. Through women's eyes. In *Conference interpreters' self-perceived status in a gendered perspective. Hermes – Journal of Language and Communication in Business* 58: 19–42. https://doi.org/10.7146/hjlcb.v0i58.111658.

Germon, Jennifer. 2009. *Gender: A Genealogy of an Idea.* New York: Palgrave Macmillan.

Hadziabdic, Emina, and Katarina Hjelm. 2013. Working with interpreters: Practical advice for use of an interpreter in healthcare. *International Journal of Evidence-Based Healthcare* 11: 69–76. https://doi.org/10.1111/1744-1609.12005.

Hall, Judith A., Julie T. Irish, Debra L. Roter, Carol M. Ehrlich, and Lucy H. Miller. 1994. Gender in medical encounters: An analysis of physician and patient communication in a primary care setting. *Health Psychology* 13 (5): 384–392.

Harrison, Wendy Cealey. 2006. The shadow and the substance: The sex/gender debate. In *Handbook of Gender and Women's Studies*, ed. Kathy Davis, Mary Evans, and Judith Lorber, 35–52. London: SAGE.

Heritage, John, and Douglas W. Maynard. 2011. After 30 years, problems and prospects in the study of doctor-patient interaction. In *Handbook of the Sociology of Health, Illness, and Healing: A Blueprint for the 21st Century*, ed. Bernice A. Pescosolido, Jack K. Martin, Jane D. McLeod, and Anne Rogers, 323–342. New York, London: Springer.

Holbrook, Sue Ellen. 1991. Women's work: The feminizing of composition. *Rhetoric Review* 9 (2): 201–229. https://doi.org/10.1080/07350199109388929.

Hu, Kaibao, and Lingzi Meng. 2018. Gender differences in Chinese-English press conference interpreting. *Perspectives* 26 (1): 117–134. https://doi.org/10.1080/0907676X.2017.1337209.

Iliescu, Cătălina. 2012. Bodily perception in female ad hoc interpreting: Romanian immigrants in contemporary Spain. *Perspectives* 20 (3): 329–343. https://doi.org/10.1080/0907676X.2012.702401.

Lee, Jieun, Moonsun Choi, Jiun Huh, and Aili Chang. 2016. Community interpreting services by marriage migrants for marriage migrants in South Korea. *Perspectives* 24 (2): 179–200. https://doi.org/10.1080/0907676X.2015.1052524.

Lehti, Lotta, Simo Määttä, and Minna Viuhko. 2021. Guiding refugee women who have experienced violence: Representation of trust in counsellors' journals. *Journal of Refugee Studies* 35 (1): 531–550. https://doi.org/10.1093/jrs/feab100.

Levinger, Miriam. 2020. Triad in the therapy room - The interpreter, the therapist, and the deaf person. *The Journal of Interpretation* 28 (1). https://digitalcommons.unf.edu/joi/vol28/iss1/5. Accessed 15 September 2021

MacDougall, D. E. 2012. Gendered discourse and ASL-to-English interpreting: A poststructuralist approach to gendered discourse and the ASL-to-English interpretive process. *Journal of Interpretation* 19 (1): 33–69. http://digitalcommons.unf.edu/joi/vol19/iss1/2. Accessed 10 September 2021

Magnifico, Cédric, and Bart Defrancq. 2016. Impoliteness in interpreting: A question of gender? *Translation & Interpreting* 8 (2): 26–45. https://doi.org/10.12807/ti.108202.2016.a03

Magnifico, Cédric, and Bart Defrancq. 2017. Hedges in conference interpreting: The role of gender. *Interpreting* 19 (1): 21–46. https://doi-org.libproxy.helsinki.fi/https://doi.org/10.1075/intp.19.1.02mag

Magnifico, Cédric and Bart Defrancq. 2019. Self-repair as a norm-related strategy in simultaneous interpreting and its implications for gendered approaches to interpreting. *Target* 31 (3): 352–377. https://doi.org/10.1075/target.18076.mag.

Magnifico, Cédric and Bart Defrancq. 2020. Norms and gender in simultaneous interpreting: a study of connective markers. *Translation and Interpreting* 12 (1): 1–17. https://doi.org/10.12807/ti.112201.2020.a01.

Maryns, Katrijn. 2013. Disclosure and (re)performance of gender-based evidence in an interpreter-mediated asylum interview. *Journal of Sociolinguistics* 17 (5): 661–686. https://doi.org/10.1111/josl.12056.

McDermid, Campbell, Brianna Bricker, Andrea Shealy, and Abigail Copen. 2021. Gendered Translations: Working from ASL into English. *Journal of Interpretation* 29 (1). https://digitalcommons.unf.edu/joi/vol29/iss1/1. Accessed 3 December 2021

Mengesha, Zelalem B., Janette Perza, Tinashe Dunea, and Jane Usshera. 2018. Talking about sexual and reproductive health through interpreters: The experiences of health care professionals consulting refugee and migrant women. *Sexual & Reproductive Healthcare* 16: 199–205. https://doi.org/10.1016/j.srhc.2018.03.007.

Nakane, Ikuko. 2008. Politeness and gender in interpreted police interviews. *Monash University Linguistics Papers* 6 (1): 29–40.

Nicodemus, Brenda S., Lori Whynot, and Poorna Kushalnaga. 2020. Insights from U.S. deaf patients: Interpreters' presence and receptive skills matter in patient-centered communication care. *Journal of Interpretation* 28 (2). https://digitalcommons.unf.edu/joi/vol28/iss2/5. Accessed 15 September 2021.

Norma, Caroline, and Olga Garcia-Caro. 2016. Gender problems in the practice of professional interpreters assisting migrant women in Australia: A theoretical case for feminist education. *Violence against Women* 22 (11): 1305–1325. https://doi.org/10.1177/1077801215623381.

Oda, Melanie, and Donna Joyette. 2001. Interpreting for the perpetrator in the partner assault response program: The selection and training process. *In The Critical Link 3: Interpreters in the Community. Selected Papers from the Third International Conference on Interpreting in Legal, Health and Social Service Settings, Montréal, Québec, Canada 22–26 May 2001.* eds. Louise Brunette, Georges L. Bastin, Isabelle Hemlin and Heather Clark, 147–161. Amsterdam: John Benjamins.

Osman, Ghada, and Claudia V. Angelelli. 2011. "A crime in another language?" revisited: Arabic-centered discourse in the Yousry case. *Translation and Interpreting Studies* 6 (1): 1–23. https://doi.org/10.1075/tis.6.1.01osm.

Pan, Jun, and Jackie Xiu Yan. 2012. Learner variables and problems perceived by students: An investigation of a college interpreting programme in China. *Perspectives* 20 (2): 199–218. https://doi.org/10.1080/0907676X.2011.590594.

Pavlidou, Theodossia-Soula. 2011. Gender and interaction. In *The sage handbook of sociolinguistics*, ed. Ruth Wodak, Barbara Johnstone, and Paul E. Kerswill, 412–427. London: SAGE.

Quinto-Pozos, David, Erica Alley, Kristie Casanova, and de Canales, and Rafael Treviño. 2015. When a language is underspecified for particular linguistic features: Spanish– ASL–English interpreters' decisions in mock VRS calls. In *Signed Language Interpretation and Translation Research: Selected Papers from the First International Symposium*, ed. Brenda Nicodemus and Keith Cagle, 212–234. Washington: Gallaudet University Press.

Roussos, Stergios, Mary-Rose. Mueller, Linda Hill, Nadia Salas, Melbourne Hovell, and Veronica Villarreal. 2010. The impact of demographics on health and health care: Race, ethnicity and other social factors. *Research in the Sociology of Health Care* 28: 217–229. https://doi.org/10.1108/S0275-4959(2010)0000028012.

Schwenke, Tomina. 2012. Sign language interpreters and burnout. *Journal of Interpretation* 20 (1): 31–54. http://digitalcommons.unf.edu/joi/vol20/iss1/7. Accessed 10 September 2021

Stone, Christopher. 2013. The UNCRPD and "professional" sign language interpreter provision. In *Interpreting in a changing landscape: Selected papers from critical link 6*, ed. Christina Schäffner, Krzysztof Kredens, and Yvonne Fowler, 84–100. Amsterdam: John Benjamins.

Valero Garcés, Carmen. 2005. Doctor-patient consultations in dyadic and triadic exchanges. *Interpreting* 7(2): 193–210. https://doi-org.libproxy.helsinki.fi/https://doi.org/10.1075/intp.7.2.04val.

Valero Garcés, Carmen, Raquel Lázaro Gutiérrez, and Maribel del Pozo Triviño. 2015. Interpretar en casos de violencia de género en el ámbito médico. In *Interpretación en contextos de violencia de género*. eds. Carmen Toledano Buendía and Maribel Del Pozo Treviño. Valencia: Tirant Humanidades.

Valero Garcés, Carmen, and Denis Socarrás-Estrada. 2012. Assessment and evaluation in labs for public service interpreting training. *International Journal of Interpreter Education* 4(2): 7–23. https://tigerprints.clemson.edu/ijie/vol4/iss2/3. Accessed 15 September 2021

Wadensjö, Cecilia. 1998. *Interpreting as interaction*. New York: Addison Wesley Longman Ltd.

Yenkimaleki, Mahmood, and Vincent J. van Heuven. 2018. The effect of teaching prosody awareness on interpreting performance: An experimental study of consecutive interpreting from English into Farsi. *Perspectives* 26 (1): 84–99. https://doi.org/10.1080/0907676X.2017.1315824.

Carmen Acosta Vicente Carmen Acosta Vicente holds a Master's Degree in Interpreting (Heriot-Watt University) and a Bachelor's Degree in Translation and Interpreting (Autonomous University of Madrid—UAM). She is currently pursuing a PhD in the Doctoral Programme in Language Studies at the University of Helsinki. Her research focuses on the role of gender in interpreting and her doctoral dissertation "The Interpreter's Gender Performance in Healthcare Interpreting—Evidence from Finnish, Spanish and English" explores how the interpreter's gender performance takes place in healthcare settings through linguistic and interactional aspects, what triggers it, and the impact it has on communication.

Cultural Competence Development in Healthcare Interpreting Training: A Didactic Proposal

Noelia Burdeus-Domingo

1 Introduction

When misunderstandings result from verbal and nonverbal behaviour, healthcare communication fades. To prevent such situations, healthcare interpreters must have attained expert levels of cultural competence, qualifying them to make optimal interpreting and mediating decisions. Evidence of this can be found in Burdeus-Domingo (2015). This exploratory study comparing the healthcare interpreting services provided in Barcelona and Montreal highlights interpreters' cultural competence as one of the most valued competences by all the parties involved in interpreted healthcare exchanges: interpreters, healthcare providers, managers of healthcare interpreting services and their users. This is because, as explained by Angelelli (2019), competency in healthcare interpreting requires the use of suitable means for sensitively engaging with individuals from diverse cultural backgrounds and lifestyle preferences, which requires high levels of socio-cultural awareness.

It is worth mentioning that, as stated by Burdeus-Domingo et al. (2021), while some academic institutions offer formal healthcare interpreting training (either at the vocational or university level), many non-academic institutions offer their own non-formal training. Frequently, the latter focuses mainly on intercultural mediation, leaving behind other aspects of the interpreting profession. Notwithstanding, training initiatives (either on interpreting or intercultural mediation) tend to be focused on diversity awareness and rarely do they explore cultures in depth, which can hinder learners' future healthcare interpreting decision-making involving cultural competence. In their professional practice, healthcare interpreters work in collaboration with healthcare providers to enable healthcare practice for allophone patients of diverse

N. Burdeus-Domingo (✉)
Valencian International University, Valencia, Spain
e-mail: nburdeus@universidadviu.com

R. Lázaro Gutiérrez and C. Álvaro Aranda (eds.), *New Trends in Healthcare Interpreting Studies*, New Frontiers in Translation Studies,
https://doi.org/10.1007/978-981-99-2961-0_4

cultural backgrounds. Sharing a common framework to build on their cultural competence would facilitate such inter-professional collaboration, leading to interventions adapted to allophone users' communicative needs.

In what follows, a didactic proposal based on the Purnell model (Purnell and Paulanka 1998/2012;Purnell 2013/2017)—which is extensively used in healthcare provider training—is presented, based on prior research on the development of cultural competence in healthcare settings. The purpose of the paper is to provide interpreting trainers with a framework for developing interpreters' cultural competence. This adds a fresh viewpoint to the field of interpreting studies, by reviewing developments in the field of transcultural healthcare.

2 Healthcare Interpreting Competences

Translation competence began to be studied in the '80s within the field of Translation Studies. Hurtado Albir (2001) describes it as the underlying systems of knowledge, skills, abilities and attitudes needed to translate. Along the same lines, Kelly (2002) defines translation competence as the macro-competence comprising the set of abilities, skills, knowledge and attitudes that professional translators possess and are involved in translation as an expert activity. PACTE (2011) describes it as a system of knowledge needed to translate. For the group, translation competence is expert knowledge, which is eminently procedural (i.e. not declarative, since, far from being theoretical, it is made up of procedures for implementing an action), formed by various interrelated sub-competences and a particularly important strategic component.

Several authors have studied translation competence in order to delimit it, describe it and list the sub-competences in which translation or interpreting learners should be trained (Bell 1991; Nord 1992; Pym 1992; Hurtado Albir 1999, 2001; PACTE 1998, 2000, 2001, 2003, 2017; Neubert 2000; Kelly 2002; EMT 2009; amongst others). One of the most popular translation competence models is PACTE's holistic model. Starting with an early version in 1998, it was progressively developed, always subjected to empirical-experimental research. Its constructs have shaped the current version (PACTE 2017) and inspired other models. PACTE's work is widely valuable within the field of translation studies and has held substantial influence on the competence model supported by the European Master's in Translation Network initiative, initiated by the Directorate-General for Translation of the European Commission with the counselling of multiple academic advisors.

Based on PACTE's proposal, Kelly's translation competence model (Kelly 2002, 2005) stands out for being specifically oriented toward shaping the curriculum design of translation programmes. Translation studies date back further than interpreting studies. For that reason, most research and reflection on interpreting competences is based on the developments of translation competence, under the framework of translation studies. Thereupon, in order to deepen the understanding of Public Service Interpreting, Abril Martí and Martin (2008) accommodated Kelly's model to this reality by describing the seven sub-competences that make up the translation competence needed for interpreting in public services (i.e. communicative and textual, cultural and intercultural, thematic, instrumental-professional, psychophysiological, interpersonal, and strategic). Burdeus-Domingo (2015) describes these seven sub-competences in the context of healthcare interpreting as follows:

- Communicative and textual sub-competence in at least two languages and cultures (different registers, dialects and varieties).
- Cultural and intercultural sub-competence: knowledge of the social and demographic phenomenon of immigration, the cultural values that affect interpersonal relationships and the concept of health.
- Thematic sub-competence: knowledge of medical practices and techniques, healthcare systems, medical discourse and terminology.
- Professional instrumental sub-competence: knowledge of the ethics of the profession.
- Psychophysiological sub-competence: self-awareness and psychophysiological skills (i.e. attention, concentration, memory, ability to analyse and reformulate…).
- Interpersonal sub-competence: social and interpersonal communication skills (i.e. ability to listen actively, assertiveness, mastery of questioning and negotiation strategies, ability to manage turn taking…).
- Strategic sub-competence: mastery of interpreting techniques.

Burdeus-Domingo (2015) explores, amongst other interpreting-related issues, the appreciation of the different competences listed above by all participants of interpreter-mediated healthcare communication. The results of this study reveal that interpreters (in both contexts) perceive instrumental-professional, interpersonal, communicative and textual, intercultural, thematic and strategic competences as essential for their professional practice. On their side, practitioners and service users highly value interpreters' communicative and cultural competencies as essential to healthcare interpreting, also cherishing interpreters' professionalism and social skills.

2.1 Cultural Competence in Translation and Interpreting Training

Olalla-Soler (2015) describes the cultural competence of translators as follows:

> The translator's abilities to effectively arrange his/her knowledge about a source culture and that of a target culture and to contrast them in relation to a cultural phenomenon perceived in a source text in order to achieve an acceptable solution in a target text. The translator's cultural competence is related to the other sub-competences that make up translation competence.

While most translation competence models recognise cultural competence as an essential competence, not all translation training programmes include courses devoted to its development (Hurtado Albir and Olalla-Soler 2016). This also applies to interpreting training programmes.

Hurtado Albir and Olalla-Soler (2016) rightly explain that culture represents a group of individuals with a common rationale, fostering a shared process of perception, judgment, attribution and decision-making encouraging certain attitudes in communication. As multilingual and multicultural communication professionals, the role of interpreters consists of facilitating understanding between healthcare professionals and users, despite their linguistic and cultural differences, making each rationale comprehensible to the other party. In this sense, cultural competence is recognised as both central and transversal for healthcare interpreting (Angelelli 2004, 2019; Pöchhacker 2007; Gustafsson et al. 2013; ISO 2014; Burdeus-Domingo 2015; Cox and Lazaro 2016; amongst others). Thus, interpreter training should entail developing expert levels of cultural competence. The reality, however, is far from resembling such a scenario: even though healthcare interpreting training programmes generally address the impact of culture in cross-cultural communication, the development of cultural competence is seldom tackled by formal instruction, possibly due to the idea that cultural competence is shaped by one's previous background and personal history. It has previously been stated that no culture could be fully covered in a single training programme (Witte 2000; Hurtado Albir and Olalla-Soler 2016). Nonetheless, as defended by Hurtado Albir and Olalla-Soler (2016), translation and interpreting programmes should include cultural content that is appropriate considering their learning objectives.

All things considered, healthcare interpreting training programmes should cover much of the same cultural content as transcultural health programmes, since cultural competence is core to both healthcare interpreting and cross-cultural communication in healthcare. However, according to the above definition, the cultural competence of translators encompasses both knowledge and abilities. Thus, it may be inferred that the ideal training actions intended to develop cultural competence in healthcare interpreting training will be able to develop both such knowledge and abilities.

3 Method

This chapter has its origins in two existing literature reviews on cultural competence in nursing: on the one hand, Shen's (2015) literature review on cultural competence models and cultural competence assessment instruments developed and published by nursing science researchers since 1982; and, on the other hand, Purnell's (2016) literature review, aiming to increase understanding of theories, models, and approaches of cultural competence in healthcare. Purnell (2016) includes (1) a list and description of the main theories, models, and approaches to developing cultural competence within nurses and other healthcare professionals, (2) a description of governmental and professional organisations' and associations' documents regulating culturally competent practices and (3) a recension of systematic reviews on the matter.

It is not the author's aim to list the different theories and models reviewed in the aforementioned publications. Instead, based on documentary research, this work examines the Purnell Model for Cultural Competence (henceforth, PMCC) to contribute with a didactic application proposal to develop cultural competence in healthcare interpreting training. This work is supported by previous publications on cultural competence development from the nursing and medical fields, which are complemented by the author's suggestions and recommendations. Having an applied didactics perspective, this work is limited to proposing a collection of activities derived from Purnell's theory and model (Purnell and Paulanka 1998/2012; Purnell 2013/2017), with the intention of contributing to the cultural competence development strategies and methods in healthcare interpreting training. Such activities are designed to be applied by interpreting learners of all languages, helping them explore different cultural issues conditioning cross-cultural communication in healthcare.

4 The Purnell Model for Cultural Competence

The PMCC was conceptualised on theories from different fields (i.e. biology, anthropology, sociology, economics, geography, political science, pharmacology, nutrition, communication, family development, and social support; see Purnell 2016, 2021). Even though it was originally designed as a framework to develop cultural competence in nursing training, it serves to frame culture on a general level within healthcare services (Marcilli 2016) and has been employed to train many healthcare professional profiles. It has also served as a framework for research on different medical fields of specialisation—e.g. gerontology (Yalçın Gürsoy and Tanrıverdi 2020), fertility (Aksoy Derya et al. 2021), palliative care (Long 2011) or public health (Phelps and Johnson 2004). Moreover, it has proved to be effective for organising curricula on the fundamentals of culture (Hudiburg et al. 2015).

According to its author (Purnell 2021), this model was based on assumptions including (but not limited to)[1] the following:

- culture has a significant impact on how people understand and relate to healthcare;
- each individual differs from the dominant culture to some extent, which should be considered to avoid stereotyping;
- all cultures share fundamental similarities and have significant differences; and
- all healthcare professionals require similar information regarding users' cultural backgrounds.

Based on the aforementioned assumptions, Purnell (2021) states that the PMCC goals are:

- to offer a framework for all healthcare providers to learn about culture;
- to describe circumstances that affect an individual's cultural worldview;
- to establish the most salient relationships of culture;
- to interconnect characteristics of culture to encourage correspondence and to enable deliberate culture competent healthcare;

[1] This list is non-exhaustive. Only some of the most salient assumptions are included. The reader is referred to Purnell (2021) for an extensive list of the assumption on which the model is based.

- to present a framework revealing human characteristics (i.e. motivation, intentionality, meaning…);
- to present a structure for analysing cultural data; and
- to consider healthcare users (individuals, families or groups) within their own ethnocultural environment.

The PMCC offers a detailed methodical framework to analyse cultures which includes reflective activities and an assessment guide to promoting cross-cultural critical thinking. Its framework comprises 12 domains around which cultural competence is developed, including overview/heritage, communication, family roles and organisation, workforce issues, biocultural ecology, high-risk behaviours, nutrition, pregnancy, death rituals, spirituality, healthcare practices, and healthcare practitioners (Purnell 2021).

As explained by Purnell (2021), the PMCC is presented in the shape of a circle,[2] stratified at different levels in the shape of rings representing, from the outside in: global society, communities, families and individuals. Inside those rings, we find a circle that is divided into 12 sections, each portraying a cultural domain serving to organise the framework of the model. Finally, in the nucleus of the model representation, we find a dark circle that represents the unknown. Underneath the circle, the graphic representation of the PMCC includes a spiky line symbolising the nonlinearity of cultural consciousness. This representation of the model is accompanied by a table[3] which, organised in the same 12 domains, provides statements that promote cultural thinking. According to Purnell (2021), this table can be adapted to (1) assess healthcare service users and (2) develop cultural competence in healthcare professionals.

5 A Didactic Application Proposal to Develop Cultural Competence in Healthcare Interpreting Training

This section presents a didactic proposal designed to provide interpreting trainers with a structured method for developing cultural competence in healthcare interpreting programmes, to better meet the communicational needs of healthcare professionals and users.

Below is a compound of training activities designed (based on the PMCC) to stimulate learners' reflection on (1) the meaning of culture, (2) the cultural backgrounds of their target communities—their similarities and differences (with respect to the local culture) and how to approach them—(3) how the healthcare culture affects and is affected by individuals' cultures and (4) how to best deal with this information to promote best practices in healthcare interpreting. All the activities

[2] The reader is referred to Purnell (2000, 2019a, b, 2021) for a clear graphical representation of the model. Direct links to these publications are available in the references section.

[3] For further information on the contents of this table, please refer to Purnell (2021).

were designed to allow interpreting learners working with any language to explore aspects of a given culture in relation to the main culture of the society where they are being trained, while reflecting on their service as interpreters (or future interpreters). Thus, the proposed activities are compatible with the special regime teaching methodology developed by the École Supérieure d'Interprètes et Traducteurs de l'Université Sorbonne Nouvelle—Paris 3 (ESIT), which has been proven applicable to healthcare interpreting programmes (see Burdeus-Domingo et al. 2021). Likewise, they are applicable both in in-person and online training courses.

The didactic proposal is divided into 12 sections, coinciding with the 12 domains of the PMCC.[4] Each section includes a brief introduction to each domain, based on Purnell (2019b), and some activities[5] that, inspired by those recommended by Purnell and Fenkl (2019, 2021) to enhance cultural competence within healthcare providers, were purposely designed to enhance cultural competence in healthcare interpreting training actions.

5.1 *Overview/Heritage*

5.1.1 Domain Description

This domain of the PMCC comprises knowledge related to the countries of origin and of residence of the participants in cross-cultural communication, as well as the effects of their cultural beliefs on healthcare. Aspects like the patient's reasons for migration, educational status, and occupation or employment status will be important information to bear in mind when interpreting, as they might condition the way they communicate. It must also be considered, however, that individuals may belong to different social groups and, therefore, have a dominant culture—shared, for instance, with another individual of the same cultural origin—and other subcultures that are specific to their social group or geographical origin, social status, etc. Interpreters will thus benefit from increasing their knowledge about the heritage of the communities they interpret for.

5.1.2 Learning Activity

This activity will serve as an introduction. It will initiate learners in the exploration of cultural differences through critical thinking, setting the mood to comparatively examine the cultures linked to their working languages through a mediating lens.

[4] May trainers need any orientation for fostering debate or critical thinking amongst any specific group of interpreting learners in the course of the proposed activities, they are suggested to refer to Purnell and Fenkl (2019, 2021).

[5] The activities have been designed to extensively cover cultural issues. However, trainers and learners must take special attention to avoid stereotyping, by always remembering that the individual's behaviours and beliefs can differ from those of their heritage culture.

Objectives

1. To promote cultural consciousness and critical thinking, avoiding stereotypes.
2. To briefly describe the cultural heritage of target communities in contrast to that one of the local community.
3. To understand how both communities' cultural backgrounds relate to each other.
4. To identify issues likely to require cultural mediation.

Task 1

The instructor proposes to fill in Table 1 with information regarding the local community:

Task 2

After brainstorming about the characteristics describing the local community, the instructor divides the group into smaller groups according to their working languages. Each group is asked to come up with a detailed description of their target community. For that purpose, they are urged to think about what makes this community different from others, especially the local community. The instructor provides them with a wider range of descriptors to cover (see Table 2).

Task 3

Each group is asked to compare both tables, thus identifying coincidences and discrepancies. For each discrepancy detected, they are asked to suggest an objective and prejudice-free explanation of such difference to the other community in their own language.

Table 1 Local community's cultural background overview table

Descriptor	Local community's cultural background overview
Beliefs and values about health and wellness	
Popular diseases and medical conditions (if any)	
Average income level (if different levels, please provide a brief description)	
Average educational level (if different levels, please provide a brief description)	
Common occupations	

Table 2 Target community's cultural background overview table

Descriptor	Target community's cultural background overview
Countries of origin	
Reasons for migration	
Frequent migration trajectories	
Beliefs and values about health and wellness	
Popular diseases and medical conditions (if any)	
Average degree of assimilation and acculturation of the community	
Average income level (if different levels, please provide a brief description)	
Average educational level (if different levels, please provide a brief description)	
Common occupations	

5.2 *Communication*

5.2.1 Domain Description

This domain includes concepts related to the concerned languages (and dialects). It involves:

- paralinguistic aspects such as volume, tone and intonation;
- relational aspects, such as eagerness to share one's ideas and emotions;
- proxemic aspects, such as spatial distancing practices;
- kinesic aspects, such as eye contact, facial expressions or body language;
- temporal aspects, such as the relationship between time and one's worldview; and
- the use of names.

5.2.2 Learning Activity

Objectives

1. To identify the local and target community's communicational patterns (in terms of paralanguage, relational issues, kinesics, proxemics, time, formality in name usage, education and health literacy).
2. To detect any communicational patterns that might be considered culturally unacceptable within the other community.
3. To consider ways of mediation amongst both cultural communicational patterns.

4. To propose best practices for interpreter's conversation management (in terms of paralanguage, relational issues, kinesics, proxemics, time, formality in name usage, education and health literacy).

Task 1

Trainees are asked to jointly complete the mind map presented in Fig. 1 to name the main features describing the communication patterns of the local community (in terms of paralanguage, relational issues, kinesics, proxemics, time and name usage). When there are no more ideas to include, the group is divided into smaller groups according to their working languages. Each group is asked to replicate the mind map, this time considering the main communication patterns of their target community.

Task 2

Considering the communication patterns described in the mind maps of task 1, each group is asked to suggest culturally acceptable practices for conversation managing between interlocutors from the local and target communities.

Task 3

Paired up with fellow learners specialising in the same target community, participants are asked to write a bilingual script for a cross-cultural healthcare situation involving a

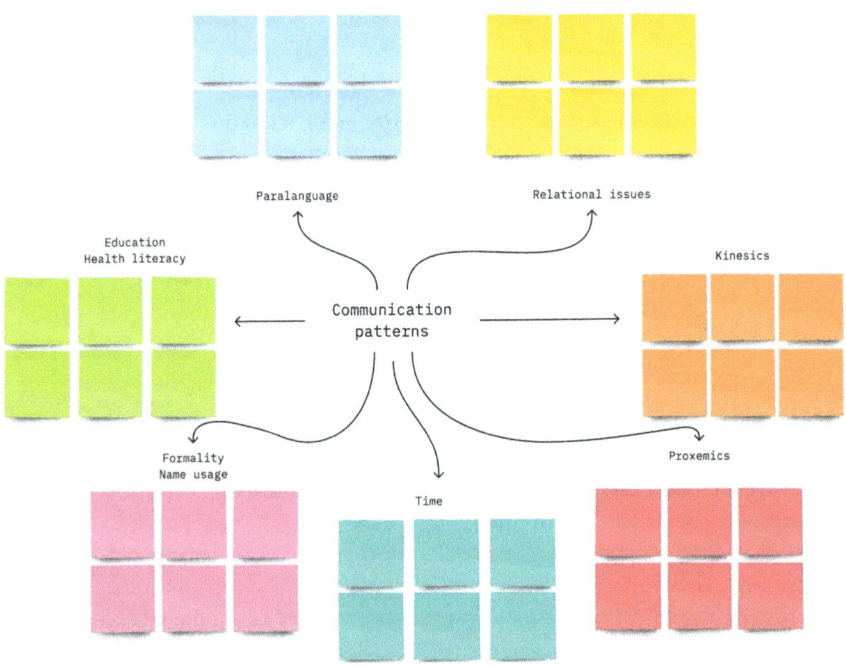

Fig. 1 Communication patterns mind map template

healthcare provider from the local community and a user from the target community. They are asked to include some of the communication patterns described in the mind maps of task 1. Once completed, each pair acts their script out, with a third learner acting as an improvised mock interpreter. This learner will have to interpret while mediating (when necessary) and managing the conversation according to the culturally acceptable practices suggested in task 2. After each performance, the group comments on the interpreter's mediation, to (1) assess how the conversation was managed, (2) highlight what communication patterns were appropriately elucidated and (3) suggest ways to improve the mediation of those that were not successfully clarified.

5.3 *Family Roles and Organisation*

5.3.1 Domain Description

This domain comprises concepts related to parentage and gender roles (within the household), as well as marriage and social status within the community.

5.3.2 Learning Activity

Objectives

1. To understand the cultural concepts of family and gender roles, marriage and social status within the local and target community.
2. To compare both cultures in regard to the terms listed above, searching for similarities and discrepancies.
3. To understand how the cultural concepts of family and gender roles, marriage and social status can hinder cross-cultural healthcare communication.
4. To set up mediation practices to convey culturally suitable meaning fostering understanding amongst the local and target culture interlocutors.

Task 1

The instructor divides the group into smaller groups. For this activity, participants are divided into groups with different fictional thinking hats: a group with the local community's thinking hat and a group per target community, wearing their respective thinking hats. All groups are asked to examine and describe the set of cultural beliefs related to the items listed below from the perspective of their group's thinking hat:

Marital/partner status—family decisions (patriarchal, matriarchal, egalitarian, depending on the decision to be made)—men/women duties—children/

teenagers do's and don'ts—family priorities—elderly roles—extended family members' roles—family status factors—extramarital children—homosexuality.

Task 2

Once each group has thoroughly outlined the cultural beliefs from the assigned perspective, the trainer suggests sharing the outcomes for each item, starting with the group with the local community's hat and then making way for the target communities'. Target communities' cultural beliefs are suggested to be presented in contrast with the local community's in order to recognise discrepancies. Learners are then encouraged, when necessary, to discuss best practices for cultural mediation dealing with the featured differences.

5.4 *Workforce Issues*

5.4.1 Domain Description

This domain embraces concepts related to autonomy, acculturation, assimilation, gender roles (within the workspace), ethnic communication styles and traditional healthcare practices.

5.4.2 Learning Activity

Objectives

1. To explore the concept of autonomy within the target community and how it relates to or differs from the local community's perception.
2. To understand gender roles in society and within the work sphere.
3. To explore the degree of integration of the target community.
4. To describe ethnic communication styles and traditional healthcare practices.

Task 1

The trainer dives learners into groups (based on their target community) and provides them all with six cards with the following titles (Fig. 2):

The trainer allocates 6 min to the first part of this task, consisting of providing ideas for each topic based on their knowledge of the target culture. When the time is up, the group discusses the ideas and fills in a group sheet describing the target community's reality concerning the issues proposed for examination.

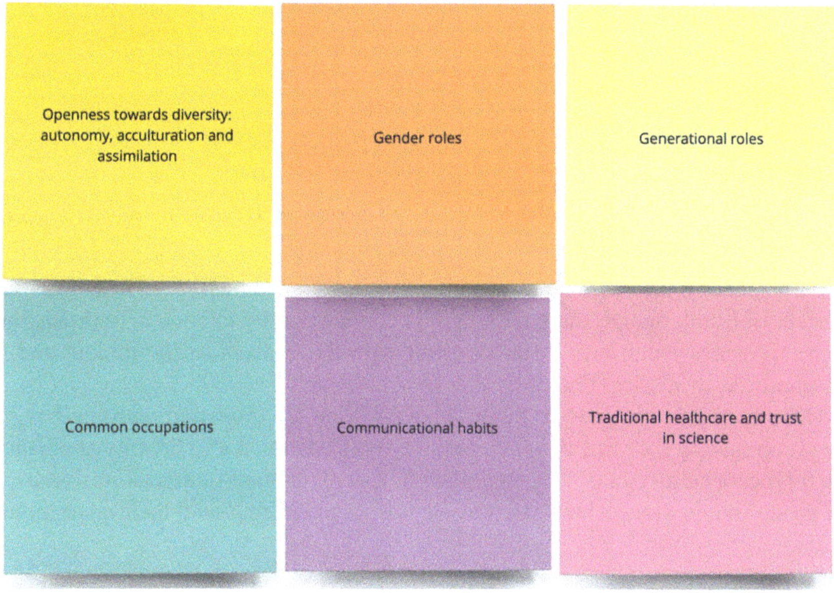

Fig. 2 Target community's workforce issues overview activity sheet

Task 2

Based on what has been discussed in task 1, each group is encouraged to debate about the most common assumptions within their target community likely to condition their daily lives in the host country and how such assumptions can hinder their integration into the local society and/or their communication within healthcare services.

Task 3

Starting from the topics discussed in task 2, in pairs, learners are asked to describe situations where such assumptions hinder communication in healthcare. If desired, they can get inspiration in real situations from their own practice as interpreters. The outcome of this activity can be discussed with the whole group in order to suggest best practices to tackle them.

5.5 *Biocultural Ecology*

5.5.1 Domain Description

This domain involves ethnic and racial issues, such as skin colour and physical differences, as well as genetic, hereditary, endemic, and topographical diseases.

5.5.2 Learning Activity

Objectives

1. To understand how ethnicity conditions the prevalence of specific health problems (due to genetics, lifestyle, environmental factors, etc.).

Task 1

In pairs (sharing the same target community), learners are asked to reflect on the concept of health, to speculate on how it is conditioned by ethnicity. To do so, the trainer provides them with a star diagram with the concept in the middle and 5 wh-questions to answer (Fig. 3).

Once each pair has provided their answers, they are discussed with the rest of the group sharing the same target community with caution not to fall into polarising stereotypes or cultural bias. If stereotypical comments or biased attitudes are detected, the group should discuss how to avoid them from interfering with their interpreting practice.

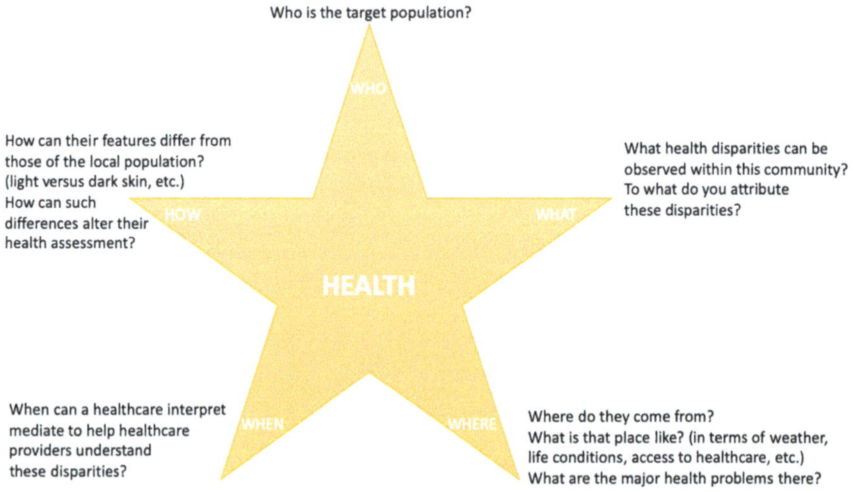

Fig. 3 Target community's biocultural ecology overview activity sheet

5.6 *High-Risk Behaviours*

5.6.1 Domain Description

This domain studies the use of addictive substances (tobacco, alcohol, recreational drugs), the lack of physical activity and the lack of safety measures—either in daily actions (using seatbelts, helmets, etc.) or in sexual intercourse.

5.6.2 Learning Activity

Objectives

1. To identify common behaviours and practices amongst the target community that might represent a risk to their health.
2. To find culturally appropriate ways to mediate when high-risk health behaviours are noticed or suspected.

Task 1

For this activity, the trainer divides the class into groups of learners working with different target communities. Each group is provided with one of the following questions:

1. In which high-risk health behaviours does your target community generally engage?
2. Does your target community do anything to control or reduce the risk? (If so, what do they do?)
3. Does your target community engage in addictive behaviours (such as smoking, drinking alcohol, taking drugs…)?
4. Does your target community use travel safety measures, such as seatbelts, helmets, etc.?
5. Does your target community engage in risky sexual practices? What types of birth control are acceptable for them?

The heterogeneous groups will discuss the culturally conditioned behaviours of each target culture.

Task 2

When the allotted time to do so is over, the trainer regroups learners according to their target community. Trainees are then asked to discuss the outcomes of each question, contrasting the behaviours of their target culture with the newfound information about other cultures. This is expected to nourish the debate on the specificities of their target community's culture.

5.7 *Nutrition*

5.7.1 Domain Description

This domain involves the meaning of food, food preferences and its usage for health promotion and wellness.

5.7.2 Learning Activity

Objectives

1. To understand the cultural concepts of nutrition.
2. To spot the main nutrition-related differences between the local and target community.
3. To understand how cultural beliefs condition the way different communities experience nutrition within different population groups (toddlers, children, teenagers, adults, elders).
4. To set up mediation practices to enhance culturally adapted nutrition practices.

Task 1

This activity is presented as a debate encouraging (self-)reflection. In groups (according to their working languages), learners are given cards with nutrition-related questions that they have to discuss in the allotted time (a few minutes per question). The questions proposed are:

1. Which foods does your target community generally eat (daily/weekly)?
2. What do they normally drink with their meals?
3. Which foods do they eat as part of their cultural heritage?
4. Do they avoid certain foods? Why?
5. Which foods do they eat and avoid when they are ill? Why?
6. Which foods are high-status foods in their family/culture?
7. Are there any foods eaten only by men, women, children, teenagers or older people?
8. How many meals do they eat per day and at what times?
9. What holidays do they celebrate and what impact do they have on the way they eat?
10. Are their food habits different on the days they work?

To conclude this task, the trainer suggests the following question to be discussed with the entire class: What will happen if, as a way to treat a physical condition or illness, a doctor suggests a certain diet without considering the explored nutritional habits? Can/should the interpreter do anything?

Table 3 Target community's nutrition habits overview activity sheet

Popular food/ingredients amongst the target community	Local popular food/ingredients rarely consumed by the target community

Task 2

Based on the information shared during the debate, each group is asked to fill in Table 3, including (1) an (extensive) list of popular food/ingredients amongst their target community, highlighting what differs from the local culture's popular food/ingredients; and (2) an (extensive) list of popular food/ingredients amongst the local community that are rarely consumed by their target community.

Task 3[6]

The trainer provides learners with a set of healthy eating food pyramids (one per group, including toddlers, children, teenagers, adults and elders) representing what is recommended in a balanced diet by local healthcare professionals. Based on the information from the previous task, learners (in groups, according to their target community) are asked to adapt the food pyramid (suggesting food selections) to their target community's food habits.

[6] Even though exceeding the functions of a healthcare interpreter—as it belongs to the practitioner to adapt diets to the tastes of users by using products and quantities adjusted to their cultures—, this kind of activity prepares learners to detect the need for mediation if dietary advice is offered to their users with no cultural adaptation.

Task 4[7]

The trainer provides learners with a copy of diet instructions commonly suggested by local healthcare providers to treat certain conditions in different age groups. Based on the information compiled in previous tasks, in groups (according to their target community) learners are asked to reflect on those instructions and detect if any mediation would be required to make sure the healthcare provider's suggestions are followed by patients from their target community. If any mediation is needed, they are asked to suggest how to approach the situation in a non-intrusive way.

5.8 *Pregnancy*

5.8.1 Domain Description

This domain concerns fertility practices and methods for birth control, as well as beliefs on pregnancy and birth.

5.8.2 Learning Activity

Objectives

1. To understand how cultural beliefs can condition fertility practices, methods of birth control, pregnancy care, birth and postpartum care.
2. To develop non-intrusive strategies to mediate in case of need in the above-mentioned contexts.

Task 1

This activity consists of an inverted brainstorming session. Trainees are asked to propose culture-related birth control, pregnancy, labour and early parenting issues in the form of questions. Those questions are expected to foster learners' internal reflection on their target cultures' habits and beliefs. The trainer will give a few examples to begin with and then ask learners to suggest new questions. The questions raised might include the following:

1. Do your target cultures have any culturally approved methods for enhancing fertility or treating infertility?
2. Do your target cultures have any prenatal beliefs or practices for (healthy) pregnancy?
3. Do your target cultures have any traditional rituals or habits practiced by pregnant women?
4. Who is present when a baby is delivered in your target cultures?

[7] Idem.

5. Do your target cultures have any particular birthing practices?
6. Do your target cultures do anything in particular after delivery?
7. Who helps with the baby after delivery in your target cultures?
8. Do your target cultures have any traditional rituals or habits practiced after birth (to increase lactation or else)?

Task 2

Trainees are divided into randomised groups. The trainer proposes some hypothetical cases (cases 1–3)[8] that groups have to reflect and debate on for a few minutes (one at a time), after which, they are asked to engage in a debate with the rest of the class to find the optimal way of dealing with each situation.

Case 1

An interpreter has been asked to intervene in the gynaecological consultations of a mother from a culture that does not allow the presence of the father at birth. The mother has experienced difficulties in labour due to a genetic abnormality of the foetus. The doctor is not aware of the cultural differences regarding the presence of the father during labour and has made a comment on this.

Should the interpreter intervene? If so, how?

Case 2

A Navajo couple with a first-time mother claims increasingly persistent and intense pain and discomfort. After an ultrasound examination, just a few days before delivery, the gynaecologist observes that the foetus is in a position that could entail a risk during labour. The doctor then suggests that the delivery should be carried out in a hospital, with adequate means to reduce the risk. When the interpreter passes the message on to the couple, the mother-to-be gets frightened and the father-to-be, not listening to reason, tries to leave the consultation, showing a nervous bound and determined attitude.

Should the interpreter intervene? If so, how?

[8] These hypothetical cases are based on different communities' cultural beliefs presented in Purnell and Fenkl (2019, 2021). May contextual information be needed, the reader is encouraged to consult publications.

Case 3
A Muslim pregnant woman always goes to her gynaecology appointments accompanied by her husband. The husband has repeatedly objected to the doctor being a man and shows little interest in issues regarding pregnancy and childbirth. The mother does not speak the language of the host country and the doctor is interested in conveying information to the mother-to-be about how the birth is going to take place. The doctor fears that cultural verbalisations and bodily expressions could lead to misunderstandings amongst healthcare practitioners during labour, which could motivate the overmedication of the mother-to-be.

Should the interpreter intervene? If so, how?

To complete this task, learners are encouraged to explore the local codes of practice in healthcare interpreting and subsequently, provide (in groups) a critical assessment of the professional expectations.

5.9 Death Rituals

5.9.1 Domain Description

This domain takes account of cultural understandings of death and bereavement, behaviours preparing for them and burial practices.

5.9.2 Learning Activity

Objectives

1. To understand death as a cultural reality and its level of acceptance as a part of life within different cultures.
2. To extensively describe the learner's target community's cultural conception of death, as well as its related behaviours and practices.
3. To develop an empathetic way to address death-related topics from a neutral but respectful perspective.

4. To be able to explain death and address death-related topics from new perspectives in a neutral but respectful manner.

Task 1

Learners are divided into groups based on their target community. Jointly, they answer the following questions, trying to provide an exhaustive description of their target community's conceptions and beliefs regarding death and death-related rituals:

1. What does death mean to your target community's culture?
2. Does your target community generally believe in an afterlife?
3. In general, do people from your target community desire to know about their own impending death?
4. How does your target community prepare for death? Do they perform any special activities?
5. What does your target community's preferred burial practices consist of? Do they include children in death rituals?
6. How soon after death do burials occur in your target community's culture?
7. What are the bereavement practices of your target community? Are they different from those of the local community? How do men and women grieve in your target community's culture?
8. What is a culturally appropriate way to address the impending death of a loved one?

Task 2

Based on the information shared in task 1, each learner individually prepares a 2-minute speech on their target culture's understandings of death and bereavement, behaviours preparing for them and burial practices to be shared (with the use of notes, if needed) with a randomised group. The information must be presented in a cautious detailed but respectful manner.

Task 3

Regrouped in randomised groups, each learner delivers the speech prepared in task 2. The rest of the group members listen carefully to the shared information and take notes, filling in the empathy mapping[9] canvas distributed by the trainer. The information collected in those empathy maps will allow learners to understand what each culture thinks and feels about death (Fig. 4).

Task 4

By turns, each learner will expose, based on the notes compiled in their empathy maps, the way an unfamiliar target community experiences death. Caution must be taken to convey accurate information in a respectful manner.

---

[9] This Empathy mapping activity is an adapted and simplified version of the proposal by Lammers (2021).

PROFILE
What culture is being presented?
ACTIONS
How should one behave when communicating with individuals from this culture?
BELIEFS
What beliefs does this culture have?
TRADITIONS
What can we expect from individuals from this culture in such circumstances?

Fig. 4 Death rituals empathy mapping activity sheet

5.10 Spirituality

5.10.1 Domain Description

This domain deals with religious practices, spiritual beliefs and sources of strength.

5.10.2 Learning Activity

Objectives

1. To understand the impact religion and other spiritual beliefs have on healthcare practices.

2. To develop cultural mediation strategies that consider religious and spiritual values.

Task 1

Divided into groups based on their target community, learners are asked to storyboard situations where religious practices and spiritual beliefs can have an impact on healthcare. If guidance is required, the instructor can share the following questions to stimulate ideas:

1. What gives strength and meaning to the lives of individuals from your target community?
2. What is your target community's main/dominant religion? Are they deeply religious?
3. What behaviours does your target community's religion encourage that could (positively or negatively) influence their health?
4. Does your target community engage in any spiritual practices to maintain their physical and mental health?

Were there to be different religious and spiritual trends amongst the target community, learners are invited to divide into smaller groups in order to work on the different realities. If the group is not large enough, one of the main religions or trends should be chosen.

Cooperative storyboarding allows awareness-raising of learners' joint understanding of how religious or spiritual realities can condition healthcare practices. It also fosters reflection on ways to overcome particular difficulties. Moreover, it serves as a way of peer tutoring, as it promotes interaction to joint problem solving by sharing different ideas.

Task 2

Each group is asked to share their story with the rest of the learners, who are encouraged to comment on the solution suggested and other possible ways of upcoming the situation, if applicable.

5.11 Healthcare Practices

5.11.1 Domain Description

This domain involves discovering and describing different healthcare practices (healing or preventive), traditional healthcare practices and beliefs, as well as potential barriers to healthcare. It reviews topics like the individual's responsibility for health, their response to pain or readiness for self-medication, as well as their views toward physical and mental illness or toward certain medical practices, such as donation and transplantation.

5.11.2 Learning Activity

Objectives

1. To detect target communities' approach to healthcare (healing or preventive).
2. To identify traditional healthcare practices and beliefs.
3. To recognise presumable barriers to healthcare.

Task 1

The trainer presents Case 4[10] to the whole group for reflection and asks learners to speculate on the reason for the narrated misunderstanding:

Case 4

A patient arrives at the emergency room of a hospital with severe knee pain after having had a work accident. He can barely walk. He is a native of a small village in Sub-Saharan Africa with low income who, due to affordability issues, has always consulted traditional medicine in his home country. He trusts much more traditional medicine than mainstream medicine, as it is grounded in his culture. He believes it to be more effective to treat psychic and psychosomatic conditions. Unable to find a traditional medicine healer within his community, he has decided to try mainstream medicine. The hospital staff asks a cleaning lady who speaks the patient's language to help with communication. After a first exploration, the doctor asks him (through the lady's mediation) to immediately get X-rays and return for consultation. The man follows the doctor's advice. When he returns for consultation, the lady gets asked to assist with communication again. Through her mediation, the patient insists on the severity of his pain. The doctor asks if he got the X-rays done and the patient confirms. There seems to be a misunderstanding. The doctor asks for the X-rays. The patient says that after getting them done, he threw them away, as they had not helped with the pain.

After a discussion of the reasons for the lack of communication, the trainer suggests a debate on what a trained interpreter would have done and how.

Task 2

The trainer asks learners to comment on whether similar situations could arrive with individuals from their target communities and encourages debate and experience sharing. If needed, the following questions can be used to further advance the debate:

1. How is health defined within your target communities? Is it perceived as the absence of illness, disease, injury, and/or disability?

[10] This hypothetical case is based on a real case reported in a previous research study (Burdeus-Domingo 2010).

2. Are mainstream healthcare services readily available to your target communities?
3. Do your target communities believe in any traditional medicine? What are its main tenets?
4. What do individuals from your target communities usually do when they are in pain? How do they express pain?
5. In what prevention activities do your target communities engage to maintain health?
6. How are people in your target communities viewed or treated when they have a mental illness?
7. What approach should the interpreter take in situations where mainstream medicine is distrusted?
8. What approach should the interpreter take in situations where mainstream medicine is not understood?

5.12 Healthcare Practitioners

5.12.1 Domain Description

This domain examines the status, consultation and perceptions of traditional and biomedical healthcare providers.

5.12.2 Learning Activity

Objectives

1. To explore the status of traditional and biomedical healthcare within the target community in order to identify if there are any preferences.
2. To explore the perceptions of healthcare practitioners both within the local and the target community and find out if (and how) they can affect cross-cultural communication).
3. To investigate the existence of any cultural beliefs conditioning patients.

Task 1

The trainer provides learners with 4 cards each. All learners of the same group (based on the target community they work with) receive cards of the same colour. They are asked to anonymously answer each question raised by the trainer (numbering their cards accordingly). The suggested questions include:

1. What healthcare providers do individuals from your target community usually consult when they are ill?
2. Are men/women likely to prefer a given profile of healthcare providers?

3. Are they likely to prefer a same-sex healthcare provider for routine health problems and/or for intimate care?
4. Do they consult any healers besides doctors and nurses? (If so, for what type of conditions are they likely to consult such healers?)

The trainer then picks the cards up again and randomly shares the answers in blocks (based on colours, representing each group). In turn, each group is invited to discuss the provided answers, trying to reach a global image of their target community and commenting on possible individual variations.

Task 2

The trainer suggests Case 5 for reflection. Trainees try to individually answer the question suggested:

Case 5

In a medical consultation requiring informed consent to proceed with a serious intervention, the patient does not seem to be understanding the message but says "yes" constantly to avoid feeling ashamed or hurting their interlocutor's or the interpreter's feelings, as is culturally expected in their culture. The interpreter understands there is a cultural difference distorting the conveyed meaning.

Should the interpreter intervene? (If so, how?).

Task 3

Based on the discussion undertaken in task 1 and following the example of task 2, in pairs, learners are asked to narrate hypothetical cases in which their target culture's beliefs can condition individuals' relationships with healthcare practitioners or distort their communication. Cases are then shared and commented on with the rest of the class, under the trainer's guidance.

6 Conclusions

Healthcare professionals' curricula and training cover cross-cultural communication issues through specific educational actions intended to develop cultural competence. This is done by applying specialised pedagogical models, which pay close attention to cultural differences in healthcare communication. Nonetheless, despite such initiatives, the advanced mastery of cultural competence remains a challenge for professionals in the field (Veliz-Rojas et al. 2019). This is hardly surprising, considering the wide variety of cultural realities that coexist today within the same society and interact in its public services. For this reason, as cross-cultural communication professionals, interpreters must provide them with culturally appropriate assistance in triad encounters.

The above notwithstanding, the development of cultural competence remains a challenge for translation and interpreting trainers, as training actions on the matter rarely tackle cultures extensively enough. In an attempt to contribute to the evolution of cultural competence teaching within translation and interpreting programmes, the present chapter has presented some didactic materials applying the PMCC (Purnell and Paulanka 1998/2012; Purnell 2013/2017) to the development of cultural competence in healthcare interpreting programmes. The aim of the proposal was to do so in light of the communicative needs of cross-cultural healthcare contexts and to align healthcare interpreter training with a common framework extensively used to train other professionals in the medical field.

As the didactic proposal has shown, applied to the training needs of healthcare interpreters, the PMCC can foster theoretical and reflective learning of the cultural differences that shape communication in healthcare contexts. Likewise, it can serve as a guide for interpreting learners toward the most salient aspects of culture and their incidence in healthcare cross-cultural communication. Reflection activities have been suggested to provide learners with the knowledge and tools needed to apply non-intrusive cultural mediation strategies, free of prejudices and generalisations. However, no theoretical instructions on what is considered a non-intrusive neutral mediation have been provided, as this exceeds the limits of cultural competence (and therefore the aim of the present work).

All things considered, due to its multidisciplinary and transdisciplinary nature, the PMCC seems a well-founded model (yet not the only one) to enhance cultural competence within the field of interpreting studies. The proposed activities may therefore help learners to develop the necessary level of cultural competence to perform holistic, culturally sensitive interpretations within cross-cultural contexts, thus promoting effective communication and fostering successful interventions in healthcare. In the long term, sharing a common frame of reference can (1) bring clinicians and interpreters closer together, (2) promote smooth communication dynamics and (3) optimise interprofessional collaboration.

While the author's extensive teaching experience supports the validity of the proposal, further research would be needed to measure its effectiveness. This could lead to its formal validation as a conclusive training strategy for healthcare interpreters, just as it is recognised to be for training healthcare practitioners.

References

Aksoy Derya, Y., S. Altıparmak, A.Ç. Karakayalı, and Z. Özşahin. 2021. Determining the Cultural Care Needs of Infertile Couples in Turkey: A Qualitative Study Guided by the Cultural Competence Model. *Journal of Religion and Health*. https://doi.org/10.1007/s10943-021-01445-w. PMID: 34687404.

Angelelli, C. 2004. *Medical Interpreting and Cross-Cultural Communication*. Cambridge: Cambridge University Press.

Angelelli, C. 2019. *Healthcare Interpreting Explained*. Oxon and New York: Routledge.

Bell, R.T. 1991. *Translation and Translating*. London: Longman.

Burdeus-Domingo, N. 2015. *Interpretación en los servicios públicos en el ámbito sanitario. Estudio comparativo de las ciudades de Barcelona y Montreal.* Ph.D. thesis. Barcelona: Universitat Autònoma de Barcelona.

Burdeus-Domingo, N. 2010. *Interpretación en los Servicios Públicos en el ámbito sanitario en la provincia de Barcelona.* Masters dissertation. Barcelona: Universitat Autònoma de Barcelona.

Burdeus-Domingo, N., S. Gagnon, S. Pointurier, and Y. Leanza. 2021. Bridges and Barriers in Public Service Interpreting Training: Instructing Non-Professional Longserving Interpreters. *FITISPos International Journal* 8 (1): 28–42. https://doi.org/10.37536/FITISPos-IJ.2021.8.1.267.

Cox, A., and R. Lázaro Gutiérrez. 2016. Interpreting in the Emergency Department: How Context Matters for Practice. In *Mediating Emergencies and Conflicts. Palgrave Studies in Translating and Interpreting*, ed. F. Federici, 33–58. London: Palgrave Macmillan.

EMT Expert Group. 2009. Competences for Professional Translators, Experts in Multilingual and Multimedia Communication. https://ec.europa.eu/info/sites/default/files/emt_competences_translators_en.pdf. Accessed 3 Jan 2022.

Gustafsson, K., E. Norström, and I. Fioretos. 2013. The Interpreter—A Cultural Broker? In *Interpreting in a Changing Landscape*, ed. Cristina Schäffner, Krzysztof Kredens, and Yvonne Fowler, 187–203. Amsterdam/ Philadelphia: John Benjamins Publishing Company.

Hudiburg, M., E. Mascher, A. Sagehorn, and J.S. Stidham. 2015. Moving Toward a Culturally Competent Model of Education: Preliminary Results of a Study of Culturally Responsive Teaching in an American Indian Community. *School Libraries Worldwide* 21 (1): 137–148.

Hurtado Albir, A. 1999. La competencia traductora y su adquisición. Un modelo holístico y dinámico. *Perspectives: Studies in Translatology* 7(2): 177–188.

Hurtado Albir, A. 2001. *Traducción y Traductología. Introducción a la Traductología.* Madrid: Cátedra.

Hurtado Albir, A., and C. Olalla-Soler. 2016. Procedures for Assessing the Acquisition of Cultural Competence in Translator Training. *The Interpreter and Translator Trainer* 10 (3): 318–342.

ISO (International Standards Organisation). 2014. ISO 13611:2014 (E): Interpreting—Guidelines for Community Interpreting (1st ed.). http://www.iso.org/iso/cataloguedetail.htm?csnumber=54082. Accessed 3 Jan 2022.

Kelly, D.A. 2002. Un modelo de competencia traductora: bases para el diseño curricular. *Puentes* 1: 9–20.

Kelly, D. 2005. *A Handbook for Translator Trainers. A Guide to Reflective Practice.* Manchester: St. Jerome Publishing.

Lammers, J. 2021. Empathy Mapping: Bridging Cultural and Linguistic Divides in International Online Education. In *International Teaching Online Symposium*, Windsor, Canada. https://scholar.uwindsor.ca/itos21/session3/session3/4/.

Long, C.O. 2011. Cultural and spiritual considerations in palliative care. *Journal of Pediatric Hematologyn/oncology* 33 (2): 96–101. https://doi.org/10.1097/MPH.0b013e318230daf3.

Marcilli, C. 2016. Assessment of cultural competence in Texas nursing faculty. *Nurse Education Today* 45: 225–229. https://doi.org/10.1016/j.nedt.2016.08.021.

Neubert, A. 2000. Competence in Language, in Languages, and in Translation. In *Developing Translation Competence*, ed. C. Schäffner and B. Adab, 3–18. Amsterdam/Philadelphia: Benjamins.

Nord, C. 1992. Text Analysis in Translator Training. In *Teaching Translation and Interpreting: Training Talent and Experience*, ed. C. Dollerup and A. Lindegaard, 39–48. Amsterdam: John Benjamins.

Olalla-Soler, C. 2015. An Experimental Study into the Acquisition of Cultural Competence in Translator Training. Research Design and Methodological Issues. *Translation & Interpreting* 7 (1): 86–110.

PACTE. 1998. La competencia traductora y su aprendizaje: Objetivos, hipótesis y metodología de un proyecto de investigación. *IV Congrés Internacional sobre Traducció.* Bellatera (Barcelona): Universitat Autònoma de Barcelona.

PACTE. 2000. Acquiring Translation Competence: Hypotheses and Methodological Problems in a Research Project. In *Investigating Translation*, ed. A. Beeby, D. Ensinger, and M. Presas, 99–106. Amsterdam: John Benjamins.
PACTE. 2001. La competencia traductora y su adquisición. *Quaderns. Revista De Traducció* 6: 39–45.
PACTE. 2003. Building a Translation Competence Model. In *Triangulating Translation: Perspectives in Process Oriented Research*, ed. Fabio Alves, 43–66. Amsterdam: John Benjamins.
PACTE. 2011. Results of the validation of the PACTE translation competence model: Translation problems and translation competence. In: *Methods and Strategies of Process Research: Integrative approaches in Translation Studies*, ed. C. Alvstad, A. Hild and E. Tiselius, 317–343. https://doi.org/10.1075/btl.94.22pac
PACTE. 2017. *Researching Translation Competence by PACTE Group*. Amsterdam: John Benjamins.
Phelps, L.D., and K.E. Johnson. 2004. Developing Local Public Health Capacity in Cultural Competency: A Case Study with Haitians in a Rural Community. *Journal of Community Health Nursing* 21 (4): 203–215. https://doi.org/10.1207/s15327655jchn2104_1.
Pöchhacker, F. 2007. *Dolmetschen. Konzeptuelle Grundlagen und deskriptive Untersuchungen*, Tübingen: Stauffenburg.
Purnell, L.D. 2000. A description of the Purnell Model for Cultural Competence. *Journal of Transcultural Nursing* 11 (1): 40–46. https://doi.org/10.1177/104365960001100107.
Purnell, L.D. 2013/2017. *Transcultural Healthcare: A Culturally Competent Approach*. Philadelphia: F.A. Davis.
Purnell, L.D. 2016. Are We Really Measuring Cultural Competence? *Nursing Science Quarterly* 29 (2): 124–127. https://doi.org/10.1177/0894318416630100.
Purnell, L.D. 2019a. Update: The Purnell Theory and Model for Culturally Comptentent Healthcare. *Journal of Transcultural Nursing* 30 (2): 98–105. https://doi.org/10.1177/1043659618817587.
Purnell, L.D. 2019b. The Purnell Model for Cultural Competence. In *Handbook for Culturally Competent Care*, ed. L.D. Purnell and E.A. Fenkl, 7–18. Cham: Springer. https://doi.org/10.1007/978-3-030-21946-8_2.
Purnell, L.D. 2021. The Purnell Model and Theory for Cultural Competence. In *Textbook for Transcultural Health Care: A Population Approach*, ed. L. Purnell and E. Fenkl, 19–59. Cham: Springer. https://doi.org/10.1007/978-3-030-51399-3_2.
Purnell, L.D., and E.A. Fenkl. 2019. *Handbook for Culturally Competent Care*. Cham: Springer. https://doi.org/10.1007/978-3-030-21946-8
Purnell, L.D., and E.A. Fenkl. 2021. *Textbook for Transcultural Health Care: A Population Approach*. Cham: Springer. https://doi.org/10.1007/978-3-030-51399-3
Purnell, L.D., and B. Paulanka. 1998/2012. *Transcultural Healthcare: A Culturally Competent Approach*. Philadelphia: F. A. Davis.
Pym, A. 1992. Translation Error Analysis and the Interface with Language Teaching. In *Teaching Translation and Interpreting*, ed. C. Dollerup and A. Loddegaard, 279–288. Amsterdam: John Benjamins.
Shen, Z. 2015. Cultural Competence Models and Cultural Competence Assessment Instruments in Nursing: A Literature Review. *Journal of Transcultural Nursing* 26 (3), 308–321. https://doi.org/10.1177/1043659614524790.
Veliz-Rojas, L., A.F. Bianchetti-Saavedra, and M. Silva-Fernández. 2019. Competencias interculturales en la atención primaria de salud: un desafío para la educación superior frente a contextos de diversidad cultural. *Cadernos de Saúde Pública* 35 (1). https://doi.org/10.1590/0102-311X00120818.
Witte, H. 2000. *Die Kulturkompetenz des Translators*. Tübingen: Stauffenberg Verlag.
Yalçın Gürsoy, M., and G. Tanrıverdi. 2020. Evaluation of Violence Against Elderly People of Different Cultures by Using The "Purnell Model for Cultural Competence". *Florence Nightingale Journal of Nursing* 28 (1): 83–96. https://doi.org/10.5152/FNJN.2020.18088.

Noelia Burdeus-Domingo holds a Ph.D. and Master in Translation, Interpreting and Intercultural Studies; a Master in Translation and Interpreting Research; and a B.A. in Translation and Interpreting. She also holds a Master and a University Expert degree in Foreign Language Teaching.

She is a Professor of the Translation and Interpreting department at the Valencian International University (Spain). From 2020 to 2023, she worked as a research fellow at the Psychology and Cultures Laboratory of Université Laval (Canada), where she previously served as a postdoctoral fellow (2017–2019). Since 2017, she has been a member of the Coordination Committee for Public Service Interpreting Access at the Capitale-Nationale (Quebec, Canada) and has collaborated with the Bank of Interpreters of the Capitale-Nationale, designing and delivering interpreting training.

Prior to this, she had been a Lecturer at the École Normale Supérieure de Lyon and Université Jean Monnet (2016–2017), a member of the research group MIRAS (Mediation and Interpreting: Research in the Social Field) (2010–2017), a research resident in the Centre d'Études Ethniques des Universités Montréalaises (2012–2013) and a doctoral researcher and interpreting trainer at the Universitat Autònoma de Barcelona (2013–2016). Her research activities focus on public service interpreting; she has published several articles in academic journals and has participated in several renowned seminars, congresses, courses and scientific dissemination events at both national and international levels.

Health Interpreting and Health Interpreter Education in New Zealand: Some Empirical Studies

Ineke H. M. Crezee and Yunduan Gao

1 Introduction

New Zealand was one of the first countries in the world to offer non-language specific health interpreter education at tertiary level when Auckland Institute of Technology offered its first Certificate course in Healthcare interpreting in 1990, in response to the findings of the Cartwright Inquiry (Cartwright 1988). The Cartwright Inquiry investigated a large-scale cervical cancer study conducted in New Zealand under Professor Green, where reportedly neither interpreters nor informed consent was used (Coney and Bunkle 1987).

New Zealand legislation has provided language access in both the health and legal settings for many years and this has been enshrined in legislation. In her doctoral thesis, Gao (2021) describes empirical research into healthcare interpreting at a large New Zealand hospital. Her thesis provides an excellent overview of legislation regarding the use of interpreters in the New Zealand health and legal settings since 1989. She writes:

> In healthcare settings, the Code of Health and Disability Services Consumers' Rights 1996 places statutory obligations on health and disability service providers to make services accessible to all consumers in New Zealand. In particular, the right to a competent interpreter is established in Right 5 (1), *Right to Effective Communication:*

I. H. M. Crezee (✉)
Auckland University of Technology, Auckland, New Zealand
e-mail: ineke.crezee@aut.ac.nz

320 Beach Road, Campbells Bay, Auckland 0630, New Zealand

Y. Gao
University of Auckland, Auckland, New Zealand
e-mail: ygao722@aucklanduni.ac.nz

Gaoxinxi District, 99 Bilin Street, Chengdu 611731, Sichuan, China

R. Lázaro Gutiérrez and C. Álvaro Aranda (eds.), *New Trends in Healthcare Interpreting Studies*, New Frontiers in Translation Studies,
https://doi.org/10.1007/978-981-99-2961-0_5

Table 1 Top five languages for telephone/video interpreting in Aotearoa New Zealand in August/September 2021

Language	Call volume		Language	Call volume	
	Aug	Sept		Aug	Sept
1. Mandarin	1576	1118	6. Persian/Farsi	212	226
2. Samoan	547	336	7. Cantonese	193	171
3. Spanish	459	423	8. Dari	150	201
4. Arabic	422	426	9. Tongan	139	125
5. Korean	215	216	10. Hindi	124	114

> Every consumer has the right to effective communication in a form, language, and manner that enables the consumer to understand the information provided. Where necessary and reasonably practicable, this includes the right to a competent interpreter (Health and Disability Commissioner (Code of Health and Disability Services Consumers' Rights) Regulations 1996) (Gao 2021, p. 11).

With regard to language access in the mental health setting, New Zealand legislation has included the Mental Health Compulsory Assessment and Treatment Act 1992 (Section 6). Gao (2021, p. 11) writes:

> Section 6 of the Mental Health Compulsory Assessment and Treatment Act 1992 not only mandates the provision of "the services of an interpreter", but also requires, "as far as reasonably practicable, that the interpreter provided is competent". However, it does not provide a definition of competence.

Gao comments that while the provision of (competent) interpreters is statutorily required in New Zealand there seems a "lack of definition of what is a competent interpreter and effective communication" (Gao 2021, p. 12).

1.1 Demand for Language Services in New Zealand

Over the years, the demand for language access services has grown exponentially, with the October Language Assistance Services Newsletter sent out on 12 October 2021 by the Ministry of Business, Innovation and Employment (2021b) showing the following ten most in-demand languages for language access services (Table 1).

As mentioned above, interpreter training has been offered in a non-language specific mode in New Zealand since 1990, however, the July 2021 Language Assistance Services Newsletter stated that by 28 July 2021, "almost 600 people registered for the Interpreter Standards Transition Package in just under three weeks". The same newsletter states that an "an analysis of the first 215 registrations from NAATI[1]" indicated that just over one third of those who registered with NAATI had "no qualifications and will be offered funded interpreter training that enables them to apply

[1] National Accreditation Authority of Translators and Interpreters.

for either Certified Provisional Interpreter or a Recognised Provisional Interpreter credential I once they have passed their initial training" (MBIE 2021a).

The fact that up to one third of those working as interpreters in New Zealand did not possess any formal qualification in interpreting is both concerning and disappointing. Especially taking into account that the use of competent interpreters in the health setting is stipulated by law and the fact that the health setting is one of the most common settings for New Zealand-based interpreters to work in.

2 Literature Review

This section will provide a brief review of the relevant literature on health interpreting and aspects of non-language specific health interpreter education such as situated learning and reflective practice.

2.1 Health Interpreting

Roat and Crezee (2015) define healthcare interpreting as "interpreting that takes place during interactions related to healthcare" (p. 237). They continue by saying that 'medical interpreting' was "a descriptor used more in the early years of the field" while 'healthcare interpreting' is a later term "recognising that the field covers interactions that are not strictly medical in nature, such as rehabilitation and mental health" (Roat and Crezee 2015, p. 237). This chapter will use the term "healthcare interpreting" for the reasons outlined by Roat and Crezee (2015).

2.2 Health Interpreter Education

For many years some interpreter educators insisted that it is sufficient to prepare student interpreters for work in the healthcare setting by teaching them medical terminology. Crezee (2013) has long argued that what student health interpreters really need is something approaching a Nursing 101 course: they need to learn about anatomy, physiology and pathology and what procedures (diagnostic and therapeutic) might be commonly implemented in the healthcare setting. Student interpreters also need to know about the healthcare system, its culture (patient-centred or family centred), referral system, and common intercultural issues. Student interpreters need to develop an awareness of not only the relevant code of ethics and code of conduct, but also develop what Dean et al. (2022) refer to as moral reasoning skills.

2.3 Non-language Specific Health Interpreter Education

Traditionally interpreter education has been language specific, allowing educators to provide feedback on student renditions. The increasing movement of migrants, refugees and asylum seekers around the world has meant this approach is now less sustainable, as interpreters are needed in a growing number of language pairs. In Australia, Hale and Ozolins (2014) report on what they term monolingual courses for language specific accreditation, while Slatyer's (2015) doctoral thesis reports on curriculum design for multilingual interpreter education. Blasco Mayor (2020) reports on the many challenges involved in organising legal interpreter training and assessment in languages of lesser diffusion in Spain. Crezee (2021) reports on the challenges of non-language specific health interpreter education in Aoteroa New Zealand, where this type of approach has been used since 1990 (Crezee 2009, 2015).

2.3.1 Situated Learning

Machles (2003, p. 23) writes "Situated learning is one of several social learning theories which imply that people learn through observation and interaction with others in a social setting" (citing Merriam and Caffarella 1991, p. 134). Situated learning is at the heart of the master-apprentice model which so successfully underpinned the training of skilled tradespeople for millennia (Evans 2009). Situated learning continues to play a major role in the education of those working with members of the public in specific settings, such as physicians, physiotherapists, speech pathologists and nurses (Gillespie and Peterson 2009). Situated learning is especially suited to helping students make effective decisions in an authentic setting (Gillespie and Peterson 2009). It facilitates learners' transition from what Lave and Wenger (1991) named legitimate peripheral participation to full participation in a community of practice.

Several interpreter educators have reported on the benefits of situated learning in interpreter education, including mock conferences (Chouc and Conde 2016; Li 2018), and shared interprofessional education involving student interpreters and health professionals (Van de Walle 2022; Crezee and Marianacci 2021; Krystallidou et al. 2018; Hlavac and Saunders 2021).

2.3.2 Self-reflective Practices and Peer Feedback

This section will look at self-reflective practices and reflections on peer feedback as an important component of non-language specific health interpreter education in New Zealand (Crezee 2021).

Self-reflection

Various interpreters and interpreter educators have explored the potential benefits of reflective practices in interpreter education. Li (2018) explored the benefits of self-assessment (SA) among a cohort of undergraduate translation majors in China. Li (2018, p. 48) writes that student-centred assessment is an important element in helping students become what she calls "self-reliant graduates, capable of judging their own work against agreed criteria and increasing their levels of competence over the course of their careers." Li (2018, p. 48) writes that student-centred assessment "requires students to critically and actively analyse and reflect on their learning progress and thus to guide new learning."

Herring and Swabey (2017, p. 27) link reflective practice by student interpreters to deliberate practice. Herring and Swabey (2017) cite Barbara Moser-Mercer's (2007) work when they write that deliberate practice requires motivation, well-defined tasks, concrete, achievable goals, feedback from others (peers or educators), analysis and reflection, and cyclical, where a sub-skill is revisited over time, systematic, and "not necessarily fun" although it should not be demotivating) (pp. 28–29).

Herring and Sawbey (2017, p. 29) write that goal setting is important, because "[p]racticing without a goal can be overwhelming because of the number of potential targets for monitoring. The ability to monitor one's performance is crucial, but this ability develops over time." They point out the important task of educators in helping student interpreters identify tasks to attend to. In the lead author's health interpreting classes, the lecturer does this by reading all self-reflections and guiding students towards specific goals, while peer feedback helps students identify specific subskills to focus on. Herring and Swabey (Herring and Swabey 2017, pp. 29–30) emphasise the importance of reflection in that it "can draw learners' attention to aspects of their Experiential Learning in Interpreter Education 31 experience they may not have consciously attended to at the time." At the lead author's university, peers often point out things students themselves had not noticed. Unfortunately, students who do not have a same-language peer in class (the 'language soloists') need to find a peer outside of the classroom who is committed to their learning and able to provide constructive feedback.

Herring and Swabey (2017, p. 27) stress the importance of normalising certain processes for students in order not to demotivate them when they write: "In spoken language interpreter education, learners will often find that their listening skills deteriorate when they begin to learn note-taking. It is helpful to normalize this process for them by framing it as a temporary regression related to adding a new sub-skill to an already complex task."

In her article, Lee (2018, p. 154) defines self-feedback as "self-review or analytic assessment based on critical listening to one's own audio- or video-recorded performance." Lee (2018, p. 154) argues that asking students to analyse their own performance "helps them to discover their weaknesses and strengths and channel their resources accordingly during training" (Van Dam 1989; Russo 1995, p. 75). Lee links this to deliberate practice (as defined by Setton and Dawrant 2016, p. 47) which she says "is critical to achieving a high level of skill mastery".

Self-reflections can be recorded in different ways: Mraček and Vavroušová (2021) asked a cohort of consecutive interpreting students to keep reflective diaries throughout their first semester. This chapter will discuss the inclusion of both weekly reflections and longer compulsory reflective written assignments in health interpreter education.

Peer feedback

Lee (2018) examined the benefits of feedback from teachers and peers in a conference interpreter training programme in Seoul. Lee found that students trusted and valued teacher feedback more than that given by language peers. Lee (2018, p. 153) divides feedback into "teacher feedback, peer feedback, and self-feedback", whereas, in the current chapter, the word feedback will be used to refer to peer feedback only. Lee (2018, p. 153) points out that "peer feedback can be provided more quickly and be more accessible than teacher feedback, and may not invoke the anxiety often associated with teacher feedback." She goes on to say that "[b]y giving feedback to and receiving it from their peers, students may develop an appreciation of what counts as quality performance (Sadler 1989) and take an active role in the management of their own learning (Liu and Carless 2006)". The program Lee (2018) reported on comprised of students and teachers all working with Korean as one of their languages—in other words, teachers were able to provide students with language specific feedback on their interpreted renditions.

Holewik (2020, p. 153) explored peer feedback and reflective practice in the context of public service interpreter training in Poland, her main focus being to explore differences between "peer feedback and self-assessment (reflection) in terms of positive aspects (strengths) and negative aspects (weaknesses) of trainee interpreters' performance in public service interpreter training." Holewik (2020, p. 154) writes that the process of reflective diary-keeping "allowed trainees to be actively involved in the learning process, recognise the value of their own work, and most importantly obtain feedback from different perspectives." This chapter will discuss student health interpreters providing feedback on interpreted renditions by same-language peers.

2.4 Authentic Health Interpreter-Mediated Interactions

There is a dearth of studies reporting on actual health interpreter-mediated interactions, as reported in the literature review section. Some previous studies present findings involving interactions which often did not involve trained interpreters. As Mikkelson writes, while some hospitals in the US and Canada started to engage paid interpreters in the 1980s, the latter were professional only in the sense that they were paid for their services, but "received little or no training and were hired based on self-reported bilingual proficiency" (Mikkelson 2020, p. 2). There is still a dearth of studies involving observations of what actually happens in interpreter-mediated health interactions, involving trained and accredited interpreters. Australia has a long history of interpreter accreditation and training, although specialist health interpreter testing[2] was only introduced more recently. Mahdavi's (2020) doctoral dissertation discusses the role of interpreters in the Australian healthcare setting. Mahdavi's work is relevant here as this chapter will present a very recent doctoral study involving health interpreters in the New Zealand setting.

3 New Zealand Studies

This section will present some New Zealand studies involving health interpreter education and observations of and interviews with participants in authentic interpreter-mediated health professional-patient interactions.

3.1 Non-language Specific Health Interpreter Education

The lead author has played a major role in developing non-language specific health interpreter education in New Zealand, becoming involved first as a student—in 1990—and then as an educator, from 1991 onwards. Health interpreter education in New Zealand was non-language specific, with English as the medium of instruction. Up until 2000, health interpreting courses were taught over two semesters, with students first receiving an introduction to interpreting, the code of ethics, note-taking and clarifying the interpreter role, before receiving a brief introduction to healthcare studies and the healthcare setting in the second semester. From the year 2000 onwards, the Auckland University of Technology (AUT) offered two advanced health interpreting courses, with students first completing an introductory course on interpreter role, ethics and practice, before moving on to the advanced health interpreting courses. Students now complete health interpreting courses as part of either a Graduate Certificate in Arts (Interpreting), consisting of four courses, or a Graduate Diploma in Arts (interpreting), consisting of eight courses. In Semester One, students learn about the body's main organ systems with associated pathology, diagnostic and therapeutic procedures. They practise short consecutive interpreting and sight translation of health documents from English into their other language. In the second semester, students learn about specialised healthcare settings, while practising simultaneous and long consecutive interpreting.

The restraints of courses taught through the English medium formed the impetus for several studies, undertaken to ensure that students' needs were met, in spite of the non-language specific nature of the courses. These studies included research on situated learning, student reflections on their own and same-language peer renditions, interprofessional learning and the challenges of understanding informal language commonly used by health professionals in Aotearoa New Zealand.

---

[2] https://www.naati.com.au/become-certified/certification/certified-specialist-health-interpreter/.

3.1.1 Situated Learning

The lead author has attempted to introduce situated learning in her courses over the decades, often hampered by a lack of technology and funding. In recent years, topical online resources such as video clips explaining medical resources can be inserted into either VoiceThread® or GoReact®, allowing students to practise interpreting while having both audio and visual cues. In the 1990s, however, interpreting practice mainly took place in language laboratories which still used tape decks and pre-recorded cassettes. Language specific interpreting exams involved frozen exam dialogues recorded by language assessors—both English speakers and speakers of Languages Other Than English (LOTEs). The lead author would borrow videos on medical topics, and show these in class, something which would see her lugging a huge trolley with a television and video recorder. She would record programmes such as RPA (Royal Prince Alfred Hospital) and Middlemore (a large South Auckland hospital) showing doctors interacting with patients, patients undergoing medical procedures and doctors explaining the outcomes to the patients. However, she was unable to provide students with the opportunity to listen to, pause and interpret based on audiovisual material.

Starting in the 1990s, the lead author would also ask hospital departments to let her have unused cardiac catheters, inhalers, insulin pens and other realia, so she could pass these around the classroom. Students in class often involved those whose languages had very limited medical terminology (Burn and Wong-Soon 2020) and being able to see and hold realia enabled these students to paraphrase concepts and equipment in their own languages. In more recent years, the lead author has ordered anatomical models of the eye, heart, lungs, kidneys and vertebrae, to pass around the classroom. Being able to touch and explore these 3-D representations of organs is an important part of situated learning. Students take part in interprofessional learning experiences with speech language therapists (Crezee and Marianacci 2021; Crezee 2015), and similar interprofessional experiences are planned with nursing students for 2022 and beyond.

3.1.2 Reflective Assignments

Health interpreting classes at AUT comprise both spoken and signed language interpreting students, where the latter are taking the courses as part of their Bachelor of Arts in New Zealand Sign Language Interpreting (NZSL).

The lack of tutors who can provide language specific feedback on spoken language students' interpreted renditions has resulted in students now needing to reflect on their own and same-language peers' recorded renditions. This has become a compulsory part of an assessment for both spoken and signed language interpreting students, since only a few learners were engaging in reflections when these were not mandated. Crezee and Burn (2019) discuss the use of reflective blogs in a multilingual, language-neutral undergraduate translation classroom, before reporting on studies where students were asked to interpret audiovisual clips showing professionals interacting with members of the public in real-life scenarios.

The New Zealand government provides additional funding for NZSL-interpreting courses and this means NZSL-interpreting students are able to receive language specific feedback from their tutors. Such feedback enables them to engage in deliberate practice, to improve on their weaknesses and further develop their strengths. Reflections written by NZSL students are commonly very specific and speak of the use of poise, facial expressions (an important feature of NZSL) and classifiers.

Reflective assignments are compulsory in the first semester of the health interpreting class, in that students must post these every week. They must also invite language specific feedback from a classmate or external language peer and reflect on that also. Students are asked to formulate what went well, and what went less well, using a reflective blog template (attached). Teaching staff check student reflections and comment on their nature and depth.

In the second semester of the health interpreting class, students must write a three-part reflective written assignment, which must cover three observed/shadowed scenarios. Two of the scenarios can be taken from the shared interprofessional education sessions with speech and language therapists, which are explained in more detail in the next section. Students are allowed to use one simulated scenario for their reflective written assignment: a video clip of an authentic bad news conversation between a gastrointestinal specialist and a patient with metastatic stomach cancer.

Students are asked to reflect on their observations by referring to the Calgary Cambridge Framework (Kurtz et al. 2003) for medical interviews, Kübler-Ross's (1973) views on death and dying and the stages of grief Dean and Pollard's (2011) Demand-Control Schema, the relevant professional codes of ethics and conduct (SLIANZ 2012; NZSTI 2013), and references to intercultural studies. Students who include the bad news clip in their reflections, often comment on the taboo nature of bad news in their culture, sometimes including the fact that health professionals may tell relatives, but not the patients themselves.

3.1.3 Interprofessional Education

From 2012 onwards, the lead author has organised shared interprofessional education sessions with a colleague who teaches postgraduate speech science students at the University of Auckland. These 3-h sessions involve speech science and health interpreting students working through two simulated real-life scenarios involving a child with possible language delay, and an adult who is being assessed for aphasia following a stroke. All postgraduate speech science students have already qualified as Speech and Language Therapists (SLTs), but may not have worked with interpreters previously. The aim of the session is to allow both student cohorts to learn by discovery and to see what issues are involved in working with interpreters in the speech language therapy setting. About half an hour before the end of the session, there is an opportunity to discuss 'take-away lessons' with members of both cohorts. Students from both cohorts are then asked to complete a short survey to see what they learned most from the session and what is needed for interpreters and SLTs to work successfully in the speech language therapy setting.

In addition to the survey, student interpreters are asked to reflect on the shared session in their reflective written assignments. Crezee and Marianacci (2021) present the findings of some of these reflections in their 2021 research article entitled *How did he say that?* The title was chosen to reflect both the importance of interpreters providing metalinguistic commentary on how something was said and the fact that a significant number of students felt it was unethical for them to provide such commentary. In 2021, student sign language interpreters argued in the post-session discussion with the speech science students that they did not feel it was appropriate for them to comment on how a Deaf individual signed something, since they might not be familiar with the person's normal idiolect when using NZSL.

3.1.4 Idiomatic Language in Health Interpreter Education

Over the years, the first author's interpreting students frequently reported a lack of understanding of idiomatic expressions in scripted dialogues. This prompted the lead author to apply for ethics approval and funding to explore students' ability to recognise and correctly interpret the informal idiomatic language used by health and other professionals (Crezee and Grant 2013, 2016, 2020). This chapter will report on the 2016 study, which involved audiovisual clips taken from real-life documentary programmes involving paramedics interacting with members of the public (Crezee et al. 2016). An analysis of the language used by the paramedics showed that they used informal language for three different reasons: to elicit information from patients or relatives and/or bystanders; to give instructions, and to present what Crezee and Grant (2016, p. 7) refer to as 'softened representations of medical reality' (SRMRs). The authors write: "Softened representations of medical reality were used to both keep patients informed as to what was happening or about to happen, but also to provide reassurance" (Crezee and Grant 2016, p. 8). The informal language proved difficult for student interpreters for two main reasons: firstly, they often did not realise that an idiomatic expression was being used, which meant they were not able to interpret it in an accurate and pragmatically equivalent manner. Secondly, student interpreters encountered intercultural issues when paramedics were addressing patients in a very informal manner, for instance by using forms of address such as 'darling', 'doll' and 'buddy'. This resulted in class discussions around such intercultural differences. Student interpreters agreed that the paramedics used such language to put patients at ease, but felt that it would be better to convey such intent by using slightly less informal forms of address, to avoid patients from cultures with a larger power distance (Hofstede 2021) from feeling offended. Such discussions in turn led the lead author to introduce the Calgary Cambridge Framework in later iterations of the health interpreting courses, with students referring to it for their reflective writing.

3.2 Authentic Health Interpreter-Mediated Interactions

This section will present some of the findings of a very recent study conducted at a large hospital in South Auckland, which combined observations with interviews with stakeholders involved in interpreter-mediated health professional-patient interviews. Middlemore Hospital, where this research was conducted, was in fact the site of the first ever health Interpreting and Translation service (ITS) established in Aotearoa New Zealand in 1991.

3.2.1 Aim

For her doctoral thesis, Gao (2021) explored healthcare interpreting services for Chinese migrant patients at Middlemore, a large hospital in Auckland, combining participant observations of interpreter-mediated interactions and individual interviews with interpreters, patients, and health professionals. Ethics approval for this study was obtained from the University of Auckland [Reference Number 023204] and the Counties Manukau District Health Board (CMDHB) [Registration Number 1033].

3.2.2 Methods

The study recruited three groups of participants from CMDHB: Chinese interpreters working in the Mandarin-English language pair, Mandarin-speaking Chinese patients, and English-speaking health professionals (doctors, nurses, physiotherapists, etc.). Informed consent was obtained from all participants prior to observations and interviews. In particular, all interpreter participants were professional interpreters employed by the Interpreting and Translation Service (ITS), CMDHB's in-house interpreting service, on a permanent or casual basis. All interpreters had received formal interpreter training of different types, primarily certificate or diploma programs in healthcare or community interpreting.

The observations consist of 18 interpreter-mediated interactions between 18 health professionals, 18 patients and four interpreters, involving 12 speciality departments or clinics (e.g., Orthopedics and Plastic and Hand Surgery). All interactions observed were consultations, where a health professional gathers information from the patient and examines the patient, before establishing diagnosis and treatment (Silverman et al. 2013). Due to ethics approval constraints, it was impossible to audio or video record the interactions. During the observations, the second author used an observation protocol she designed to collect data, notably the setting and participants, demands the interpreters encountered, and controls they employed (Dean and Pollard 2013). The interview data consist of 23 individual, semi-structured interviews with eight interpreters, nine patients, and six health professionals. Patient interviews were in Mandarin, health professional interviews were in English, and interpreter interviews were in Mandarin (six) or English (two) of participants' choice. Data were collected using an interview guide, designed to elicit in-depth accounts of participants' experiences and perceptions of healthcare interpreting services. Interviews (except one patient interview) were audio recorded and transcribed by the second author to facilitate data analysis. The study used Braun and Clarke's (2006, 2013) thematic analysis method to analyze the observation and the interview data, separately.

3.2.3 Key Observation Findings

Guided by Dean and Pollard's (2013) demand-control schema (DC-S) as a work analysis tool, thematic analysis of observations revealed a set of demands that arose for interpreters mediating health professional-patient interactions. Observations also found that in responding to these demands, interpreters employed various controls before and during the assignment, termed by Dean and Pollard (2013) as pre-assignment and assignment controls.

The most frequently observed demands were interpersonal, pertaining to the interactions between participants. A major subcategory identified was a common *lack of briefing* from health professionals, which posed challenges to interpreters preparing for assignments and interpreting accurately and effectively. This finding was surprising as it contravenes interpreters' professional conduct (NZSTI 2013) and best practice guidelines for DHB health professionals (Waitemata DHB 2020; Auckland DHB 2015). To address this interpersonal demand, interpreters employed a pre-assignment control—*direct preparation*—by interacting with the patient and family in the waiting room before the consultation. This control not only enabled proper preparations as interpreters were informed of the purpose of the consultation and patient conditions but also contributed to rapport building.

Interpersonal demands also typically occurred when health professionals did not speak in reasonable segments, or when patients failed to provide coherent answers. These demands, relating to the *communication styles* of patients and health professionals, presented a challenge to interpreting accuracy and effectiveness. To cope with health professionals' long speech segments, interpreters used two assignment controls: *asking for clarifications* and *negotiating communication flows* (interrupting speakers to interpret a shorter segment). The two controls reflect the 'discourse management skills' that NAATI (2016) expects of an interpreter, representing good practice which ensured comprehension and accuracy in interpreting. In light of patients' incoherent and ungrammatical discourse, interpreters exercised the assignment control of *re-seeking information*. While serving to keep the interaction on track, this control took the interpreters outside their professional role. Another assignment control, *improving speech*, was also observed in response to the same demand—an interpreter re-packaged the patient's speech coherently and grammatically to facilitate health professional comprehension. However, this intervention seemed deviant from the accuracy principle as it altered the style of the original discourse.

Other notable interpersonal demands were observed that placed significant challenges for interpreters to practice within their professional role, one that prohibits advising and cultural mediation. These demands first included *role understandings and expectations*, manifest in occasions where the patient or the family sought the interpreter's advice on treatment options. These demands also included those relating to *cross-cultural aspects*, particularly regarding the relatively higher level of family involvement in patient care in the Chinese culture than that in New Zealand (Mehta 2012). Observations captured an active participation of some Chinese families, which manifested when they requested the interpreter to withhold delivering cancer diagnosis to the patient, and when they attempted to sign the patient consent form. In relation to this role- or culture-related interpersonal demands, a typical control was *maintaining role boundaries* (assignment), whereby interpreters refrained from providing medical advice and from obliging the family who expected to hide cancer diagnosis from the patient. Other notable controls were *explaining the health system* and *explaining cultural differences* (assignment), observed when the patient and the family sought medical advice, and when the patient expected the family to sign the consent form. Despite being discouraged in the New Zealand context, interpreters' cultural mediation efforts seemed desirable as the efforts helped patients and their families better understand the New Zealand health system and culture.

Environmental demands (i.e., demands related to the characteristic of the healthcare settings) also appeared frequently, with healthcare terminology constituting a major demand subcategory. Interpreters in this study encountered a range of specialized terms across clinical settings, including both English terms (e.g., 'collapsed lung', 'rheumatologist') and terms from Traditional Chinese Medicine (e.g., '正骨' [chiropractic]). Typical controls involved were pre-assignment ones, specifically the resources that interpreters brought in by virtue of their *education* and *experience* in the interpreting and medical fields. The findings support Crezee's (2021) argument that health interpreting education should strive to help students develop a solid health knowledge base. This study further suggests that this knowledge base should encompass the traditional medical culture of migrant patients (e.g., the Chinese medical culture), in addition to the Western biomedical culture.

Paralinguistic demands (i.e., those pertaining to factors affecting the quality of utterances) and intrapersonal demands (i.e., those pertaining to how the interpreter felt) were also observed. Paralinguistic demands primarily included patients' *regional accents*, which presented challenges to comprehension and effective communication. As a typical response, interpreters exercised the assignment control of *asking for clarifications* to ensure accurate interpreting. Intrapersonal demands observed were *physical and cognitive strains*, which arose from the physically and cognitively taxing nature of interpreting in healthcare, and *psychological stress*, which stemmed from safety concerns when infectious diseases were involved. While not being directly observable, two pre-assignment controls—*experience* and *personal attributes* (i.e., physical, cognitive, and psychological endurance)—supposedly came into play. Interpreters may also have employed *self-care* as a post-assignment control, as the interpreter interviews revealed.

3.2.4 Key Interview Findings

Interview findings from the study centred around several themes relating to ethical and professional practice in healthcare interpreting from the perspectives of interpreters, patients, and health professionals.

These themes first included the interpreter's role and role boundaries. A commonly shared perception among participants was that interpreters were communication aids, facilitating interactions between patients and health professionals through message transfer. This perception matches the fundamental interpreter role prescribed by interpreters' professional ethics and conduct (NZSTI 2013). Additionally, interpreters were perceived by some patients as the 'walking stick' and 'close friends', and by some health professionals as members of the healthcare team.

Interviews further suggested that interpreters undertook various tasks outside their prescribed role, due to what patients and health professionals expected, and what interpreters themselves believed. This article focused on two tasks that constituted deviations from interpreting ethics and practice standards—providing emotional support and giving advice. The two interventions are discouraged in the New Zealand context, as they may deviate from the requirements of 'clarity of role boundaries' and 'impartiality' (NZSTI 2013). However, interviews revealed that emotional support to patients (expressions of empathy, care, and concern) was commonly practised by interpreters, and expected by both patients and health professionals. This was mainly because all three parties generally believed that emotional support played a vital role in patient care, especially for patients with major health issues. However, there were concerns as to if interpreters had sufficient expertise to provide emotional support, especially in forms of giving comfort or counselling. Regarding giving advice, interviews suggested that patients may expect medical advice (e.g., on treatment and medication). Health professionals may also expect advice, specifically cultural advice (e.g., how to handle cross-cultural communication breakdowns) and advice on if the patients' speech was coherent and honest. Interestingly, while interpreters would generally avoid providing patients with medical advice, they appeared willing to comply with health professionals' requests. This illustrates how institutional expectations may impact the interpreter's role (Davidson 2000).

A second theme this study explored concerned interpreter impartiality. Interpreters showed overall confidence in maintaining impartiality, namely "remain[ing] unbiased throughout the communication" (NZSTI 2013, p. 2). Some spoke of a dilemma about whether to remove the displeasing content or tone in health professionals' messages to prevent conflicts, or to adhere to the impartiality principle. Dilemmas may also occur due to patients' expectations for medical advice and emotional support, and health professionals' expectations for cultural advice, as discussed previously. Interpreters also reportedly showed bias for no good reason, according to patients and health professionals. These included biased attitudes towards patients, demonstrated by omitting patients' questions and talking to patients impatiently. Despite this, patients and health professionals largely considered the interpreters they had engaged to be impartial.

A third theme explored was the accuracy requirement in healthcare interpreting. Interviews with interpreters revealed numerous demands interpreters frequently experienced and the controls they tended to use to ensure interpreting accuracy, most of which were corroborated by the observation findings. A demand reported but not observed concerned interpreters' *feelings of sympathy*, an intrapersonal demand that might result in interpreters deviating from the impartiality requirement. Reported controls that were not captured by observations notably included *ongoing self-learning* (post-assignment), and *note-taking* (assignment). Another key finding from the interviews was confusion among interpreters over the notion of accuracy. Notably, interpreters appeared confused as to whether accuracy means preserving the original style and tone, in addition to the meaning of messages, as the NZSTI (2013) Code of Ethics and Code of Conduct (Codes) are not explicit about this. This finding suggests that the NZSTI (2013) Codes need to expatiate on the notion of accuracy, explicitly indicating register and style, as well as pragmatic intent (Crezee et al. 2020; Teng et al. 2018; Hale 2014).

Another key theme revealed by the interviews related to cross-cultural communication between Chinese patients and New Zealand health professionals. Interviews found that Chinese patients tended to experience difficulties navigating the New Zealand medical system and culture. Patients tended to be frustrated with the referral system in New Zealand, particularly the long waits for specialist care, and medical examinations. Additional to system-related factors, cultural differences appeared to be another potential source of communication breakdowns. First, interpreters and health professionals noted that family members of Chinese patients tended to actively participate in consultations, as corroborated by and discussed in the observation findings. This result might reflect the collectivist orientation of some Chinese migrants impacting patient-health professional interactions (Mehta 2012; Meyer 2016). Relatedly, health professionals noted that Chinese patients tended to be inactively involved in the decision making process, probably influenced by a relatively more hierarchical healthcare culture the patients were from, compared with the mainstream biomedical culture which encourages shared decision making (Silverman et al. 2013). Communication might also break down due to a stigmatising attitude of some patients towards mental health issues. In responding to cross-cultural communication breakdowns, interpreters generally reported resorting to cultural mediation which was documented in observations, primarily by explaining the health system and cultural differences. Patients and health professionals, by contrast, tended to expect faithful interpretations only, without distortions or omissions.

Finally, this study explored participants' notions of healthcare interpreter competence, within the framework of NAATI's (2016) competency standards. This framework is relevant as the New Zealand government is implementing NAATI credentialing for all New Zealand public service interpreters, including healthcare interpreters. Among the eight competencies in the NAATI (2016) standards, several were considered important by participants in this study. These were: thematic competency (paralleling the competency termed *healthcare knowledge and terminology* this study identified); transfer competency (paralleling the *information transfer* competency);

service provision competency, specifically interpersonal skill (paralleling the *interpersonal competency*); and ethical competency (paralleling the competency termed *professional ethics*). Due to reasons of space, this chapter does not detail the findings relating to this theme.

4 Discussion

Health interpreter education in Aoteroa New Zealand celebrated its 30th birthday in 2021, a milestone that passed unnoticed as the pandemic shifted our focus to moving all interpreter education and assessment online. 2021 was also the year the Interpreting and Translation Service at Middlemore Hospital celebrated its 30th anniversary, so it is fitting that this chapter comprises a short summary of the findings of a doctoral research study conducted at that hospital.

Non-language specific interpreter education has become more accepted in countries outside of Aotearoa New Zealand. This form of interpreter education continues to present challenges, and is sometimes hampered by a lack of funding for research. In addition, the complexities of applying for ethical approval often impinge on teaching staff research, supervision and teaching workloads. This is a shame, since it is very clear that the findings of interpreter education research inform continuous improvements made to the way in which health interpreter education and assessment are shaped.

Studies focusing on student interpreters' ability to recognise and interpret idiomatic language provided new insights into this often-overlooked aspect of health interpreter education. Research on shared interprofessional education involving student health interpreters and speech and language therapists have resulted in interesting discussion about the interpreter role, and the need for interpreters to work closely with speech and language therapists. This includes the need for a briefing where both interpreters and SLTs explain their expectations, and where SLTs clarify the aim and purpose of the assessment. The findings of the research on shared interprofessional education have also provided the impetus for further sessions, this time involving student nurses undertaking health assessments.

Research on the benefits of reflective written assignments reported on here is continuing to uncover the benefits of teaching students about the Calgary Cambridge framework (Kurtz et al. 2003) and asking students to reflect on intercultural issues, which may impact on interpreting in the health setting. Admission to a hospital often triggers deeply held cultural beliefs about health, which may impact on how patients respond to suggested procedures and investigations.

The research on reflective written assignments has also shown the benefits of familiarising students with Dean and Pollard's (2011) Demand-Control Schema (DC-S) in the compulsory interpreter role, ethics and practice course, which all health interpreting students must complete before taking the health course. DC-S offers students a robust framework for analysis when reflecting on challenges (demands) and controls used to address those challenges. The benefits of DC-S as a framework for analysis are also apparent from Gao's (2021) doctoral study, where she used it to analyse pre-, peri- and post-assignment demands observed when she was present at real-life health interpreter-mediated interactions.

5 Concluding Remarks

This chapter has provided a brief history and overview of health interpreter education in Aotearoa New Zealand, as well as a look at what actually happens when (trained) interpreters interact with health professionals and patients in the healthcare setting.

This chapter has reviewed some of the findings of research involving student health interpreters in the Aotearoa New Zealand setting. Some of these studies were made possible using the funding which was available up to recently, while others involved time rather than money, thereby demonstrating that research can be carried out 'on a shoestring' (to use an informal expression) if absolutely necessary. Such studies were inspired by student needs (e.g., the need to understand informal idiomatic language in health dialogues) and are essential in the authors' efforts to continue to improve health interpreter education.

Gao (2021, p. 252) suggests that the main implications for interpreter education of her doctoral study include the importance of using (semi-)authentic materials, role-plays involving health professionals, and field observations. Studies such as Mahdavi's (2020) and Gao's (2021) are crucial for health interpreter educators, being all the more important because they involve professional (trained) interpreters following a professional code of ethics (NZSTI 2013), something that has not always been the case in earlier studies, as pointed out by Gao (2021).

Healthcare interpreters play a crucial role in helping facilitate access to the healthcare system, and it is essential that they are adequately trained and prepared for this role. The authors hope that the research reviewed in this chapter may contribute to improving both health interpreting and health interpreter education.

References

Auckland District Health Board. 2015. *Interpreters*. https://assets.ctfassets.net/uszvm6pv23md/2ZsIUXUPXyvzeSMPefnywS/5cce520d04a59936fc53b42888bd2498/Interpreters.pdf.

Blasco Mayor, M. J. 2020. Legal translator and interpreter training in languages of lesser diffusion in Spain. In *Interpreting in legal and healthcare settings: Perspectives on research and training*, ed. E. Ng, and I. Crezee, 133–164. John Benjamins. https://doi.org/10.1075/btl.151.06bla.

Braun, V., and V. Clarke. 2006. Using thematic analysis in psychology. *Qualitative Research in Psychology* 3 (2): 77–101. https://doi.org/10.1191/1478088706qp063oa.

Braun, V., and V. Clarke. 2013. *Successful qualitative research: A practical guide for beginners*. Sage.

Bunkle, P. and Coney, S., 1987. An unfortunate experiment at National Women's Hospital. Metro June, 47–65.

Burn, J.A., and H.N. Wong-Soon. 2020. Interview with Samoan-English specialist mental health interpreter Hoy Neng Wong Soon. *International Journal of Interpreter Education* 12 (2): 63–67.
Chouc, F., and J. M. Conde. 2016. Enhancing the learning experience of interpreting students outside the classroom. A study of the benefits of situated learning at the Scottish Parliament. *The Interpreter and Translator Trainer* 10 (1): 92–106. https://doi.org/10.1080/1750399X.2016.1154345.
Committee of Inquiry into Allegations Concerning the Treatment of Cervical Cancer at National Women's Hospital and into Other Related Matters. 1988. The report of the Committee of Inquiry into Allegations Concerning the Treatment of Cervical Cancer at National Women's Hospital and into Other Related Matters. Government Printing Office: New Zealand.
Crezee, I. 2009. Development of the interpreting profession. In *Interpreting in New Zealand: The pathway forward*, ed. D. Clark and C. McGrath, 75–79. Office of Ethnic Affairs.
Crezee, I. 2013. Introduction to healthcare for interpreters and translators. *John Benjamins*. https://doi.org/10.1075/z.181.
Crezee, I. 2015. Semi-authentic practices for student health interpreters. 7 (3): 50–62. https://doi.org/10.12807/ti.107203.2015.a04.
Crezee, I. 2021. Non-language-specific health interpreter education: Challenges and solutions. In *Global insights into public service interpreting: Theory, practice and training*, ed. R. Moratto, and Defeng Li, 185–201. Routledge. https://www.routledge.com/Global-Insights-into-Public-Service-Interpreting-Theory-Practice-and-Training/Moratto-Li/p/book/9781032053189.
Crezee, I., and J. A. Burn. 2019. Action research and its impact on the development of pragmatic competence in the translation and interpreting classroom. In *The Routledge handbook of translation and pragmatics*, ed. R. Tipton, and L. Desilla, 355–372. Routledge. https://doi.org/10.4324/9781315205564.
Crezee, I., and L. Grant. 2013. Missing the plot? Idiomatic language in interpreter education. *International Journal of Interpreter Education* 5 (1): 17–33.
Crezee, I., and L. Grant. 2016. Thrown in the deep end: Challenges of interpreting informal paramedic language. *Translation and Interpreting* 8 (2): 1–12. https://doi.org/10.12807/ti.108202.2016.a01.
Crezee, I., and L. Grant. 2020. An Achilles' heel? Helping interpreting students gain greater awareness of literal and idiomatic English. *International Journal of Interpreter Education* 12 (1): 43–61. https://tigerprints.clemson.edu/ijie/vol12/iss1/5.
Crezee, I., and A. Marianacci. 2021. 'How did he say that?' Interpreting students' written reflections on interprofessional education scenarios with speech language therapists. *The Interpreter and Translator Trainer* 1–20. https://doi.org/10.1080/1750399X.2021.1904170.
Crezee, I., E. Zucchi, and S. Jülich. 2020. Getting their wires crossed: Interpreters and clinicians' expectations of the role of the professional interpreters in the Australian health context. *New Voices in Translation Studies* 2020 (23): 1–30. https://mro.massey.ac.nz/handle/10179/15924.
Davidson, B. 2000. The interpreter as institutional gatekeeper: The social-linguistic role of interpreters in Spanish-English medical discourse. *Journal of Sociolinguistics* 4 (3): 379–405. https://doi.org/10.1111/1467-9481.00121.
Dean, R., and R. Pollard. 2011. Context-based ethical reasoning in interpreting. *The Interpreter and Translator Trainer* 5 (1): 155–182. https://doi.org/10.1080/13556509.2011.10798816.
Dean, R., and R. Pollard. 2013. *The demand control schema: Interpreting as a practice profession*. CreateSpace.
Dean, R., V. Samar, and D. Maffia. 2022. Are two heads better than one? Interpreting students' moral reasoning skills. *International Journal of Interpreter Education* 14 (1).
Evans, R. 2009. The guilds and apprenticeships. In *A short history of technical education*, vol. 2022. Technical Education Matters.
Gao, Y. D. 2021. Exploring healthcare interpreting for Chinese immigrants in Aotearoa New Zealand: Current practices and stakeholder perspectives. Doctoral thesis, The University of Auckland.

Gillespie, M., and B. L. Peterson. 2009. Helping novice nurses make effective clinical decisions: The situated clinical decision-making framework. *Nursing Education Perspectives* 30 (3): 164–170. https://journals.lww.com/neponline/Abstract/2009/05000/Helping_Novice_Nurses_Make_Effective_Clinical.7.aspx.
Hale, S. 2014. Interpreting culture. Dealing with cross-cultural issues in court interpreting. *Perspectives* 22 (3) : 321–331. https://doi.org/10.1080/0907676X.2013.827226.
Hale, S.B., and U. Ozolins. 2014. Monolingual short courses for language-specific accreditation: Can they work? A Sydney experience. *The Interpreter and Translator Trainer* 8 (2): 217–239. https://doi.org/10.1080/1750399X.2014.929371.
Health and Disability Commissioner (Code of Health and Disability Services Consumers' Rights) Regulation. 1996. https://www.legislation.govt.nz/regulation/public/1996/0078/latest/DLM209080.html.
Herring, R., and L. Swabey. 2017. *Experiential learning in interpreter education*. St: Catherine University.
Hlavac, J., and B. Saunders. 2021. Simulating the context of interpreter-mediated social work interactions via interprofessional education. *Linguistica Antverpiensia, New Series-Themes in Translation Studies* 20: 186–208.
Holewik, K. 2020. Peer feedback and reflective practice in public service interpreter training. *Theory and Practice of Second Language Acquisition* 2 (6): 133–159.
Hofstede, G. 2021. *Hofstede insights*. https://www.hofstede-insights.com/.
Krystallidou, D., C. Van De Walle, M. Deveugele, E. Dougali, F. Mertens, A. Truwant, and P. Pype. 2018. Training "doctor-minded" interpreters and "interpreter-minded" doctors: The benefits of collaborative practice in interpreter training. *Interpreting* 20 (1): 126–144. https://doi.org/10.1075/intp.00005.kry.
Kübler-Ross, E. 1973. *On death and dying*. Routledge.
Kurtz, S., J. Silverman, J. Benson, and J. Draper. 2003. Marrying content and process in clinical method teaching: Enhancing the Calgary–Cambridge guides. *Academic Medicine* 78 (8): 802–809. https://journals.lww.com/academicmedicine/Fulltext/2003/08000/Marrying_Content_and_Process_in_Clinical_Method.11.aspx.
Lave, J., and E. Wenger. 1991. *Situated learning: Legitimate peripheral participation*. Cambridge University Press.
Lee, J. 2018. Feedback on feedback: Guiding student interpreter performance. *Translation and Interpreting* 10 (1): 152–170. https://doi.org/10.12807/ti.110201.2018.a09.
Li, X. 2018. Self-assessment as 'assessment as learning' in translator and interpreter education: Validity and washback. *The Interpreter and Translator Trainer* 12 (1): 48–67. https://doi.org/10.1080/1750399X.2017.1418581.
Liu, N., and D. Carless. 2006. Peer feedback: The learning element of peer assessment. *Teaching in Higher Education* 11 (3): 279–290. https://doi.org/10.1080/13562510600680582.
Machles, D. 2003. Situated learning. *Professional Safety* 48 (9): 22–28.
Mahdavi, M. 2020. The role of interpreters in healthcare in Australia. Doctoral thesis, Victoria University. http://vuir.vu.edu.au/.
Mehta, S. 2012. Health needs assessment of Asian people living in the Auckland region. Northern DHB Support Agency. https://www.ecald.com/resources/publications/healthneeds-assessment-of-asian-people-living-in-theauckland-region-2012/
Mental Health (Compulsory Assessment and Treatment) Act. 1992. https://www.legislation.govt.nz/act/public/1992/0046/latest/whole.html.
Merriam, S., and R. Caffarella. 1991. *Learning in adulthood*. Jossey-Bass.
Meyer, E. 2016. *The culture map: Decoding how people think, lead, and get things done across cultures*. PublicAffairs.
Mikkelson, H. 2020. Development of the medical interpreting profession in the US: A case study. In *Handbook of research on medical interpreting*, ed. I. E. T. de V. Souza, and E. Fragkou, 1–25. IGI Global. https://doi.org/10.4018/978-1-5225-9308-9.ch001.
Ministry of Business, Innovation and Employment. 2021a. *Language assistance services newsletter*.

Ministry of Business, Innovation and Employment. 2021b. *Language assistance services newsletter*.
Moser-Mercer, B. 2007. Skill acquisition in interpreting: A human performance perspective. *The Interpreter and Translator Trainer* 2 (1): 1–28. https://doi-org.ezproxy.auckland.ac.nz/10.1080/1750399X.2008.10798764.
Mraček, D., and P.M. Vavroušová. 2021. Self-reflection tools in interpreter training: A case study involving learners' diaries. In *Changing paradigms and approaches in interpreter training*, ed. P. Šveda, 229–247. Routledge.
NAATI. 2016. *Skills and competencies for interpreting*. NAATI. https://www.naati.com.au/information-guides/descriptors-for-interpreting/.
New Zealand Society of Translators and Interpreters. 2013. *NZSTI code of ethics and code of conduct*. New Zealand Society of Translators and Interpreters. http://www.imiaweb.org/uploads/pages/102.pdf.
Roat, C., and I. Crezee. 2015. Healthcare interpreting. In *The Routledge handbook of interpreting*, ed. H. Mikkelson, and R. Jourdenais, 211–225. Routledge. https://doi.org/10.4324/9781315745381.
Russo, M. 1995. Self-evaluation: The awareness of one's own difficulties as a training tool for simultaneous interpretation. *The Interpreters' Newsletter* 6: 75–85.
Sadler, D.R. 1989. Formative assessment and the design of instructional systems. *Instructional Science* 18: 119–144. https://doi.org/10.1007/BF00117714.
Setton, R., and A. Dawrant. 2016. *Conference interpreting: A complete course*. John Benjamins.
Silverman, J., S. Kurtz, and J. Draper. 2013. *Skills for communicating with patients*. Taylor and Francis Group. http://ebookcentral.proquest.com/lib/auckland/detail.action?docID=4742673.
Slatyer, H. 2015. Multilingual interpreter education curriculum design and evaluation. Doctoral thesis, Macquarie University.
SLIANZ. 2012. *Code of ethics*. Sign Language Intertpreters Association of New Zealand. https://slianz.org.nz/working-with-interpreters/code-of-ethics-code-of-conduct/.
Teng, W., J.A. Burn, and I. Crezee. 2018. I'm asking you again! Chinese student interpreters' performance when interpreting declaratives with tag questions in the legal interpreting classroom. *Perspectives* 26 (5): 745–766. https://doi.org/10.1080/0907676X.2018.1444071.
Van Dam, I. M. 1989. Strategies of simultaneous interpretation. In *The theoretical and practical aspects of teaching conference interpretation*, ed. L. Gran, and J. Dodds, 167. Udine: Campanotto Editore.
Van De Walle, C. 2022. Involving foreign-language speaking simulated patients in medical interpreter training: A qualitative study. *Translation and Interpreting* 14 (1).
Waitemata DHB. 2020. *Guidelines for working with interpreters*. Waitemata District Health Board, eCALD Services. https://www.ecald.com/resources/cross-cultural-resources/guidelines-for-working-with-interpreters/.

Ineke Crezee is New Zealand's first full Professor of Translation and Interpreting and in 2020 was made an Officer of the New Zealand Order of Merit for services to translator and interpreter education over the past 30 years. She is a practising translator, interpreter and educator. Her book, "Introduction to Healthcare for Interpreters and Translators" was released in 2013, and was followed by iterations aimed at interpreters and translators working with Spanish, Chinese, Korean, Japanese and Arabic as their working languages, while a Russian adaptation is forthcoming and a Turkish one is in progress. She has published widely on health interpreting and interpreter education.

Yunduan Gao trained as a conference interpreter, graduating with a Master of Arts in Language Studies (Translation and Interpretation) from the City University of Hong Kong before moving to New Zealand to continue her studies. She completed a Master of Professional Studies in Translation at the University of Auckland, focusing on bibliometric studies, before completing her PhD on authentic interpreter-mediated interactions between New Zealand health professionals and Mandarin Chinese-speaking patients, also at the University of Auckland. Yunduan Gao is a certified interpreter and translator, full member of the New Zealand Society of Translators and Interpreters (NZSTI).

A Diachronic Assessment of Healthcare Interpreting: The Western Cape, SA as a Case in Point

Harold Lesch

1 Introduction

In the recent past, the global migrant population has significantly increased, and as a result, large numbers of foreign-born persons do not speak the official language(s) of the host countries where they reside. This is also the case in more affluent countries on the African continent. Obviously, these language barriers will affect the quality of healthcare available to these individuals. South Africa is currently home to approximately 4.2 million migrants from the region, excluding the total number of refugees in the country. This addition of foreign cultures further diversifies the multilingual nature of the South African society itself. (https://southafrica.iom.int/, press release, 2020).

This compounded linguistic reality has put an extra burden on the healthcare sector during the covid pandemic as it is not only fellow citizens, but also migrants that become a social liability for the healthcare sector. From a public health perspective, urban development and migration patterns in the province have changed the linguistic environment of public healthcare and the welfare of patients and intercultural communication for efficient healthcare service necessitated an appropriate language mediation intervention. Inevitably, health authorities face difficulties with designing and implementing city-wide public health interventions, because the burden of disease and healthcare demands within the City of Cape Town population has changed relatively rapidly.

Medical doctors are trained but also practise in a limited number of languages. However, limited the number, using more than one language eases the load of a language barrier between the service provider and the user of that service. Unfortunately, in a country with no less than eleven official languages, and a growing migrant

H. Lesch (✉)
Department Afrikaans and Dutch, Stellenbosch University, Cape Town, South Africa
e-mail: hlesch@sun.ac.za

R. Lázaro Gutiérrez and C. Álvaro Aranda (eds.), *New Trends in Healthcare Interpreting Studies*, New Frontiers in Translation Studies,
https://doi.org/10.1007/978-981-99-2961-0_6

population, it is inevitable that the average public hospital healthcare practitioner will be confronted with a language barrier that necessitates the use of a language mediator. Effective communication is seriously hampered by these language barriers, and they pose special challenges to service delivery, particularly in the healthcare sector. On-site interpreting is considered most conducive to enable effective communication, but it is not always practical and financially viable to employ on-site interpreters for all the possible language combinations in a developing context.

Diseases do not differentiate between races, cultures, and languages or linguistically disadvantaged people in multicultural and multilinguistic societies. It also holds true for a diverse context like the Western Cape, South Africa, which is home to refugees and migrants whose mother tongues are not the mainstream language and who rely on translation and interpreting services to receive information related to their healthcare. As one can gather, miscommunication and language barriers do not only exist in communication with tourists or immigrants, but also among the country's own inhabitants. Miscommunication may lead to misdiagnosis and/or incorrect usage of medication, which in turn may have devasting results for aftercare and the succession of a (successful) medical procedure.

Against this backdrop, the objective of this paper is to trace the practice of healthcare interpreting in the recent past in Cape Town and its immediate surroundings. This paper is set as follows: firstly, the research question is stated; the context is then provided; a relevant literature review follows; instances and types of healthcare interpreting are provided as manifested in the Cape Metropole with their challenges; thereafter a discussion follows with a conclusion.

2 Research Question

Language policy played a crucial role in the transformation of SA and consequently the implementation of an interpreting service to support it. The underlying question is what the development of healthcare interpreting in Cape Town and its immediate surroundings is as the country has since the dawn of democracy had a multilingual language policy in place. It is important that in a multilingual society with a divisive past, but also with rather low literacy levels among patients of public health facilities, the question is how much progress has been made to bridge the language barriers that exist between healthcare professionals and patients.

3 Context

South Africa is a multilingual democracy that was established in 1994.[1] The most spoken languages in the Western Cape province are Afrikaans (41.4%), isiXhosa (28.7%), and English (27.9%). Despite the parity of esteem of the three official languages in the Western Cape, research suggests that English and Afrikaans continue to dominate the system, to the detriment of isiXhosa. English is quite often the preferred language of healthcare providers, as more than 80% of healthcare interactions occur across language and cultural barriers.

With the language legislative framework in place on national and provincial levels, it implies in theory that the implementation thereof should be applied. The language policy and translation and interpreting policy are supposed to link up with one another; however, in practice, this is not necessarily the case in the public sector, especially when it comes to interpreting services.

Although an efficient interpreting service can add to quality healthcare, full-time permanent healthcare interpreters are uncommon. The Red Cross Hospital on the Cape Flats took the brave step in the mid-1990s to rather appoint non-professional interpreters when two nursing ancillary positions became available to assist with intercultural communication and improved healthcare. The Department of Health was responsible for compensating these healthcare interpreters.

As we do not have a long history of interpreting, the training facilities have apparently been taken up by non-governmental organisations such as the now-defunct National Language Project that focussed on the language needs of the community in and around Cape Town. Groote Schuur, linked to the Medical Faculty of the University of Cape Town, also later recruited staff members that often took on the role as ad hoc interpreters and trained them by means of a course (Saulse 2010: 53–57). Since 2003, Stellenbosch University, situated just outside of Cape Town, has taken the leading role in training interpreters in the Western Cape in a joint effort with the provincial Department of Health and Department of Arts and Culture.

Language planning and policies in SA are very progressive and are considered among the best; however, one may argue that language policy implementation is still a very problematic area. A considerable segment of the population in the surrounding areas of Cape Town is still in the grip of a language barrier in healthcare. This is also enhanced by the several dialects of the indigenous languages which are not necessarily mutually intelligible. The decision for a multilingual language policy

[1] The reality of the situation in South Africa is that there are eleven official languages, 10 indigenous languages, and English. The 11 official South African languages include English, Afrikaans, Ndebele, isiXhosa, isiZulu, Swati, Southern Sotho, Sepedi, Tsonga, Tswana, and Venda. From these languages, each province has its own official languages. In the case of the Western Cape province, the aim of its language policy is to ensure the equal status and use of the three official provincial languages, namely Afrikaans, English, and isiXhosa. In general, most South Africans speak at least two languages—typically English and one of the other languages. Currently, there is an ongoing debate about whether Afrikaans, with its roots from the Netherlands, should be classified as an indigenous language. The indigenous African languages, in turn, have several dialects that are not necessarily mutually intelligible.

was encouraged by a need to heal the divisions of the past and to build a united and democratic country whereas consideration regarding the practical implementation was less of a problem during the multi-party negotiations (Lesch 2009: 61–63).

Internal migration patterns into the province have a significant influence on healthcare provision. The first, the internal migration pattern, is a major migration stream from the Eastern Cape province of young isiXhosa-speaking households moving from the rural area. As a result of this stream, isiXhosa has recently surpassed English as the second-most spoken language (at home) in the Cape Unicity. The second migration pattern is a smaller migration stream of foreign Africans who speak a range of languages that are new to the country and equally pose a challenge for efficient communication in public spaces.

Cape Town Unicity's health system is managed and funded concurrently by the Western Cape provincial health system and the South African national health system. The overall three-sphere health system is characterised by three levels of healthcare, namely primary, secondary, and tertiary care (Department of Arts and Culture 2003). Briefly, this system which starts with the patient's first point of contact with a general practitioner or nurse is known as **primary**-based healthcare and is offered in facilities such as mobile clinics, community health centres, and day hospitals that are situated nearest to the patient's place of residence. However, if the patient cannot be immediately treated or cured, the patient is referred by a primary-level doctor to a **secondary-** (or district-) level facility. These facilities comprise general hospitals and are larger in terms of the size and expertise of their operations. In the third place, patients who suffer more serious or urgent health problems, including emergencies, will be referred to **tertiary**-level medical facilities. These include academic and centralised hospital departments where patients undergo further observation. These facilities also tend to fulfil the functions of both primary- and secondary-level care to a certain extent.

Tertiary-level facilities do not only accommodate patients inside municipal and provincial government spheres, but also at national and even continental levels. Although tertiary-level facilities comprise all the expertise and operations of primary- and secondary-level facilities, emphasis is placed on primary-level facilities: the province expects approximately 90% of the patients who seek medical attention at a nearby clinic to be treated effectively at that level (Cole et al. 2003). Healthcare interpreters are needed at all three levels of healthcare facilities, including in mental health facilities. The mental healthcare institutions make provision for psychological healthcare for patients where diagnosis and intervention occur primarily through communication between the patient and the healthcare practitioner. Once again, communication across the language barriers is a necessity.

4 Literature Review

With reference to healthcare, most medical staff in Cape Town and its immediate surroundings are Afrikaans- and English-speaking, with patients speaking a large variety of the official and unofficial African languages (Schlemmer and Mash 2006; Van den Berg 2016). In the Western Cape province, most patients are Afrikaans-speaking, creating tension when isiXhosa-speaking staff members cannot communicate with them or vice versa. A number of research studies and literature reviews on healthcare interpreting have been performed in South Africa—mostly in the Western Cape (Monroe and Shirazian 2004; Karliner et al. 2007; Leanza 2007; Lesch 2007; Saulse 2010; Brink 2014; Benjamin et al. 2016; Claassen et al. 2017; Maphumulo and Bhengu 2019; among others) and in the rest of the country (Levin 2006; Schlemmer and Mash 2006; Pfaff and Couper 2009; Ndachi 2014; Khumalo 2015; among others) where the problem is most pertinent. The researchers were unanimous in their opinion that there certainly is a great need for improved interpreting services in the South African healthcare sector.

Where healthcare interpreters are available, the state health services appear to be superior, particularly for monolingual isiXhosa speakers. Most facilities are, however, without officially trained interpreters (Williams and Bekker 2008)—even though limited inroads have been made in the recent past.

The demand for language services between clinicians and patients is critical in mental health as diagnosis takes place primarily by communication and miscommunication associated with a language barrier could be detrimental. Inexperienced and untrained interpreters can influence the outcome of the diagnosis as "(a)ccess to good quality health care should be available to all, and not just to those fluent in the dominant language. Various consequences and difficulties for patients and clinicians are created due to the language barrier, with linguistic and cultural communication difficulties cited as two of the most common barriers to health care access" (Hagan et al. 2020: 2). Ad hoc interpreting arrangements are often the norm, and these situations can cause both distress for the clinician and humiliation to the patient. This situation leads to the conclusion that "psychiatrists experience numerous difficulties in conducting their work due to the language barrier. This has an impact on their ability to provide adequate mental health care to patients. There is a need for better language services to ensure that everyone that seeks mental health care can receive the same level of care (…)" (Hagan et al. 2020: 1).

5 Consolidating Interpreting in Healthcare

This section serves to give an overview of the development and challenges in healthcare interpreting in the Western Cape.

5.1 Healthcare Interpreting at the Turn of the Century

Popular communication efforts to navigate between languages and to address the language barriers in healthcare include linguistic code-switching and code-mixing, the use of a few basic lexical items in the patient's language, and impromptu strategies, such as the help of family members, hospital security guards, and nurses to take on the role as informal interpreters. Our context in this regard is no exception in the development of healthcare interpreting. Research conducted by the now-defunct National Language Project (NLP) during the early 1990s (Ntshona 1999) indicated that there is a crisis in the health service in and around Cape Town, where the primarily English- or Afrikaans-speaking healthcare providers and the isiXhosa-speaking patients do not understand one another. Only limited inroads have been made in this regard. Crawford (1994) confirmed that interpreting in Western Cape hospitals is done on an ad hoc basis and had no status attached to it at the time. Likewise, the NLP concluded that there were no professional interpreters and isiXhosa-speaking nurses, and general assistants are often called upon. It was also not strange to call on the family members of the patient to interpret. This situation was confirmed by the Emzantsi report (Cole et al. 2003: 28–29) which was compiled for the Western Cape Department of Arts and Culture. In the report, the authors (Cole et al. 2003) note that the major demand for interpreting services is clearly in the Department of Health, where the need for health workers and patients to understand one another is often a matter of life and death.

With reference to interpreting, the aforementioned report confirms the following at the turn of the century with reference to intercultural communication in healthcare (Cole et al. 2003: 29): the main need is for interpreting between isiXhosa (i.e., an indigenous African language) speakers and non-isiXhosa health workers; there are no *official* interpreters in healthcare; and the primary interpreter resources are nurses, nursing assistants, auxiliary staff, and volunteers from the community which were entirely informal (thus non-professional interpreters). It was also highlighted in the report that the requirements for healthcare interpreters are more than just being able to speak two languages, as they should also acquaint themselves with the relevant vocabulary and terminology. The linguistic challenges also include the fact that the informal isiXhosa interpreter may not always have *adequate knowledge of English or Afrikaans*, whereas others complain that they do not always understand the "deep rural isiXhosa" of some patients. These extra-linguistic characteristics for the healthcare interpreters include, among others, that the interpreter needs to show empathy and sensitivity for the doctor-patient relationship, including an awareness of the role and responsibility of the interpreter in this relationship network. The interpreter should further have the ability to deal with patients' socio-cultural perspectives of health problems.

The report recommends, among others, that healthcare interpreters require both professional language practitioner training and specific health interpreting training (Cole et al. 2003). The healthcare interpreters are likely to be newly recruited language practitioners, possibly with limited experience in interpreting, who should provide an interpreting service for patients with a limited educational background. However, language is not the only challenge for these liaison interpreters in a new multilingual dispensation as we are confronted in a developing context like the Western Cape, South Africa with huge gaps in education levels. Consequently, the role of the liaison interpreter is to facilitate communication between a public service provider (i.e., healthcare professional) and a user of that service who does not share the same language or culture. Nevertheless, the point of departure is a recognition that the problem of communication between these two parties is not *simply a matter of language or culture*, but that the challenge is deepened by the fact that they are separated by a wide gap of power. This power discrepancy between a medical professional and the lay client/patient necessitates the services of an interpreter for effective communication. Benjamin et al. (2016: 73) echoes this by stating the following:

> There has been a longstanding call to employ trained interpreters to address language barriers in health care in South Africa. The international literature shows that while trained interpreters can be effective, the existing sophisticated models of upper-income countries are expensive and contextually inappropriate for low-resource settings like South Africa. In community interpreter models, members of the community are given brief training in interpreting; these models have a number of potential advantages for our context (...)

Even though these shortcomings have been identified and the legislative framework is in place to enhance effective language practice, it is not always possible for the powers that be to address all public needs at the same time as these needs must compete for budget with other pressing needs.

5.2 *Telephone Interpreting to the Rescue*

In 2010, a private telephone interpreting initiative was launched by Folio InterTel as the first telephone interpreting service to address the dire need for interpreting services in the healthcare system. Folio InterTel provides a remote telephonic interpreting service for healthcare in the Western Cape. The reasons given for telephone interpreting to be considered in a developing context like the Western Cape include, among others, that it is less expensive than on-site interpreters. In certain parts of the country, access to on-site interpreters is not guaranteed and it is not viable to have on-site interpreters in all the language combinations, particularly not when the additional languages spoken by immigrants are also taken into account (see https://www.folio-online.co.za/#folio-intertel for more information).

After three years of inception (2013), the number of interpreters working on a freelance basis at Folio InterTel varies between 130 and 150 and a telephonic interpreting service in 37 different languages[2] is available. As the interpreting needs

[2] These languages include African, Middle Eastern, Asian, and European languages. The South African languages include Afrikaans, Ndebele, Sepedi, Sesotho, Setswana, Siswati, Tsonga, Venda, isiXhosa, and isiZulu. Other African languages that are also catered for include Arabic, Bemba, Igbo, Lingala, Luo, Oromo, Shona, Somali, Swahili, Tonga, Tshiluba, Yoruba, Chichewa, Kirundi,

are regionally bound, the highest number of requests for isiXhosa is because the service is implemented in the Western Cape as isiXhosa is one of three official languages of the Western Cape province. If the service expands to another province, e.g., KwaZulu-Natal, the language requested most may well be isiZulu (Brink 2014: 59).

After the initial pilot phase[3] in October 2010, the implementation of the service commenced the following year (Brink 2014). Brink (2014: 58–59) confirmed that the greatest need for telephone interpreting was for isiXhosa (see Ntshona's remark again above), but immigration to the province also necessitated other requested languages spoken on the continent which include Swahili, Shona, French, and Chichewa.

There are arguments both for and against telephone interpreting. Due to the considerable demand for interpreters and the inability of hospitals to employ permanent interpreters, the use of telephone interpreters in a developing context could also serve as a solution for the language impasse. In her study, Brink (2014: 82–85) concluded that the InterTel service work adequately despite some problems. These included the quality of the telephone equipment used in the hospitals or clinics being suspect as the telephone interpreters could not hear the other parties involved in the interpreting session clearly. A concern is of course the fact that it is underutilised, seemingly due to poor facilitation and a lack of awareness and training—not due to shortcomings in the service itself.

One should consequently guard against poorly recruited and trained interpreters and, ultimately, an inadequate service within the context, if the interpreting service is not to be jeopardised. In accordance with Kelly (2008: 35–48), one is of the opinion that to enhance the interpreting service, sufficient emphasis should be placed on adequate training and the desired profile of the ideal candidate for these freelance interpreters, and balancing interpreting methodology and practice, as telephone interpreting as a genre has its own challenges. An academically sound training model grounded in research-based training for skilled and equipped telephone interpreters should be the foundation, i.e., training that is underpinned by justified academic principles and that exceeds the master-apprentice training model or mere generic principles.

Against this background, I concur with Brink (2014: 85–87) that efficient training should be provided for recruits which should exceed the obvious, such as vocabulary, professional conduct, and confidentially (Kelly 2008: 254). However, specific attention should be paid to the absence of visual elements that remain some of the key concerns in telephone interpreting. Telephone interpreters should therefore be trained to interpret intonation, tone of voice, and other speech cues to compensate

Amharic, and Malagasy. The Middle Eastern and Asian languages offered are Arabic, Lari, Mandarin Chinese, Japanese, and Thai. European languages include French, Italian, German, Portuguese, Russian, and Spanish. One should add that the French speakers referred to here are primarily French-speaking migrants from former French colonies on the African continent.

[3] The pilot phase was launched at four hospitals and one clinic, namely Tygerberg and Karl Bremer hospitals (Cape Town); Swartland Hospital (Malmesbury); Worcester Hospital; and De Doorns Clinic. It ran for three months.

for the lack of visual elements. The latter is, however, not unique to our context but is a universal reality for remote interpreting.

5.3 On-Site Interpreting in Healthcare

Apart from the private initiative of telephone interpreting in healthcare, on-site interpreting is the norm. As mentioned earlier, the healthcare sector in the Western Cape is characterised by primarily Afrikaans- and English-speaking doctors, who do not understand isiXhosa-speaking patients. In order to bridge this language gap, ad hoc interpreting services (i.e., the interpreter received no or very limited training; see also Antonini et al. 2017: 4–8) are often employed. These interpreting services are often rendered by family members of a patient, nurses, or at times even by porters or cleaners. Part of the limited inroads that have been made was to train these individuals.

Healthcare interpreting has the following main objectives: to empower patients and to improve healthcare service delivery (Lesch and Saulse 2014). These can be considered the key intended positive effects for making an interpreting service available. However, because the aforementioned ad hoc interpreters lack training in interpreting methodology and practice, they often tend to distort communication, which impacts negatively on the quality of the healthcare services that are delivered. This consequent lack of quality in healthcare can be directly related to the quality of the interpreted product that the interpreter renders. In short, apart from the main intended effects of improved healthcare, the interpreting service unfortunately also has unintended effects such as the utilisation of non-professional, ad hoc interpreters. This situation affects the service as those interpreters do not possess the necessary professional status. The effects further include (Lesch and Saulse 2014: 14–15): that the interpreting service is unorganised; that the interpreters are not visible enough; that patients are under the impression that the interpreters are constantly available; that there is a waiting period for interpreters and a shortage of interpreters; that interviews and visits are to be rescheduled due to the unavailability of interpreters; and that healthcare practitioners are not informed about how to use interpreters.

Lesch and Saulse (2014) also confirm that ad hoc interpreters lack training in interpreting methodology, and it leaves them vulnerable to distort communication, which impacts negatively on the quality of the healthcare that the patient receives or the informed consent as incorrect information is transferred. However, the effect of the presence of the interpreter is still perceived as positive by the patients. The consequent lack of quality in healthcare can therefore be directly related to the quality of the interpreting service as there is a dialectical relationship between effective communication and the healthcare service provided.

Discourse in healthcare is generally characterised by a profound imbalance of power between the doctor and patient. With the turn to the new political dispensation, Crawford (1994) focuses on hospitals in Cape Town and mentions that the patient is generally subjected to the medical gaze which establishes the patient as a body which can be probed and diagnosed while the doctor occupies the position of power.

What cannot be seen or measured in this way is discounted or relegated to the margin of the irrelevant or the irrational (Crawford 1994: 2). For Crawford (1994: 2), this was more than just a politically correct statement at the time. She continues:

> All discourse involves questions of who can speak and who must be silent; which stories can be told and which can be suppressed in terms of the relations of power in a specific social formation. In biomedical discourse the patient's story is not central - the doctor asks closed-ended questions in relation to a body of knowledge that is not accessible to the patient in order to make a diagnosis. (Crawford 1994: 2)

In essence, the doctor holds the master narrative. This is also true in the event of patients who operate within the same language and cultural paradigm as the doctor—but more so in the case of intercultural communication. The lines of power run from the doctor to the patient. With the huge discrepancy between the educational levels complemented by the language diversity, this is especially true in SA. Consequently, the healthcare interpreter has a major role to play to level the discursive field in this regard.

5.4 *Role-Shifting—An Unintended Effect*

In accordance with the legislative framework in place, healthcare interpreting has as its main objectives to empower patients and to improve healthcare service delivery. These can be considered the main intended (positive) objectives for making an interpreting service available (Lesch 2020: 19). Quite often the consequent lack of quality in healthcare can be directly related to the quality of the interpreted product that the interpreter renders. What is less obvious is that non-professional, ad hoc interpreters can also have unintended effects.

Healthcare professionals sometimes have expectations that interpreters cannot meet. In a study entitled "Health workers: idealistic expectations versus interpreters' competence" conducted by Feinauer and Lesch (2013) in three tertiary hospitals in Cape Town, interpreters were expected to declare in writing that they assisted the medical investigator to explain the information in consent forms for parents of the specific patients and volunteers on HIV therapy. It was expected from the interpreters to declare that the patients fully understood the content of the relevant document and that all their questions were satisfactorily answered. To answer the question satisfactorily is one aspect but it is indeed a tall order for the interpreters to declare that the patients fully understand the content. Their study indicated, however, that the interpreters did not fully understand the information that they had to explain. None of the interpreters interviewed wanted to sign the agreement certifying that they explained the information of the trial in the patient's mother tongue and that the patient understood it. In this study, it was discovered that the interpreters had to take primary responsibility for conveying the message. Taking the level of education of the interpreters into account, it seems impossible for them to explain the medical procedures so that the patients can make an informed decision. In their paper, Feinauer and Lesch (2013) concluded that the interpreters are set up for failure when they are confronted with this task and related documents. Plain language, which is accessible to these non-professional interpreters, is accordingly advisable.

Fine (2001: 19–21) describes plain language as clear, understandable, accessible, and user-friendly. It is therefore understandable and in formative language, with a clear and well-organised structure, a clear and user-friendly layout and design for written materials, using visual back-up when speaking, and an appropriate and user-friendly tone and body language when speaking. For readers and listeners at different levels, plain language means writing and speaking at a level that most people can understand. A plain language approach to communication for the sake of interpreting in a multicultural context requires that the service provider (professional) think of plain language as part of effective communication. It should be borne in mind that there are degrees or levels of plainness. From an interpreter's perspective (more so if they are non-professional or semi-qualified interpreters), it is advisable to receive the source text in plain language to limit the mental effort of the interpreter and to guarantee easy mental accessibility.

The obvious effect of making interpreters, whether unqualified or poorly qualified, available in healthcare is to assist with better service delivery, especially if there is a communication impasse. However, it also results in unintended effects of which one is to shift the responsibility from the healthcare professional to the interpreter. One can stipulate this as an unintended and undesirable effect of the interpreting service. Interpreters at three tertiary hospitals in the Western Cape were consulted. Regarding the interpreters' qualifications, none had a tertiary education and not all had even completed their secondary education. Regarding their training and experience, the interpreter at Tygerberg Hospital (TBH) had no formal training, but was a nursing auxiliary, who was later just shifted into an interpreting "position". The two interpreters at Red Cross Hospital (RXH) have been performing interpreting duties for at least seven years. They are full-time interpreters and had training for two years on an ad hoc basis from a non-governmental organisation. Apart from language and interpreting skills, they also had some training in counselling. These two presented themselves in a very professional manner. The three interpreters at Groote Schuur Hospital (GSH) had been doing interpreting at this hospital for the past two years but were doing interpreting on an ad hoc basis at the hospital for at least ten years before that, even though their job title was that of "cleaner". When they were appointed as interpreters, they underwent some relevant basic training for six weeks.

If these interpreters were to be confronted with this task, the ethical response would be to withdraw from the assignment unless they are supplied with a document written in plain language or, preferably, have a healthcare provider with them doing the actual explanation. This behaviour of shifting the responsibility to the interpreter, and putting in writing the effectiveness of the message, was never intended but is an unintended observable effect of the availability of the interpreters and borders on unethical behaviour.

5.5 *Interpreting in Mental Health*

Language and communication are essential for quality mental healthcare and are a vital, yet complex, part of the diagnostic and treatment process. According to Hagan et al. (2020: 1), the ad hoc interpreting arrangement in South Africa concerning mental healthcare can result in embarrassment and misery for both the clinician and the patient. Within the context of mental healthcare, effective communication is vital for the correct diagnosis of the patient. It is essential that the mental health worker and the patient should clearly understand one another. It is only then that the patient would be able to clearly communicate their symptoms to the clinician and the clinician would be able to diagnose them correctly. As a result, the patient can better adhere to the treatment and reach the desired outcomes (Hagan et al. 2020: 1).

The above sentiment is also echoed by Swartz et al. (2014) who note that language is at the centre of mental healthcare. High-income countries often have sophisticated interpreter services, but in low- and middle-income countries as in SA there are not sufficient professional services—let alone interpreter services. Task-shifting is often suggested as a solution to the problem of scarce mental health resources. The large diversity of languages, aggravated by wide-scale migration, has implications for the scale-up of services. Swartz et al. (2014) suggest that it would be useful for those who are working in mental healthcare to be creative and to explore and report on issues of language and how these have been addressed. To address the essential presence of an interpreter in healthcare settings in the broader Cape Town area, a team of relevant experts consisting of colleagues involved with interpreting training and language-specific expertise, psychology, and psychiatry was put together to train interpreters specifically for mental healthcare. Fifteen first-language isiXhosa speakers with a formal matric, i.e., the highest school-leaving certificate, were recruited as healthcare interpreters on a contract basis under the Expanded Public Works Programme (EPWP). They underwent a short course training programme of three days. The 15 trainees had to interpret between the indigenous isiXhosa and English. After their training, they were placed at mental health wards or institutions in the Western Cape. Two years after the training, the Department of Health successfully motivated for the establishment of permanent posts, and 11 interpreters were officially employed as interpreters.

Benjamin et al. (2016: 74) emphasise the importance of interpreting and they state that healthcare interpreting is a complex process, even more so in the case of mental healthcare, which aims to achieve a workable understanding which can be useful during the clinical encounter. It requires of the language intermediary more than merely knowing two languages but also to be aware of the cultures involved, the specialist terminology, and emotional vocabularies. Words and decontextualised phrases or sentences do not often translate easily or accurately, particularly medical jargon, and cultural matters and other sociopolitical differences (such as level of education) are conveyed through language in the form of proverbs, emotional undertones, and humour. These can be challenging even for experienced interpreters.

Benjamin et al. (2016: 74–75) continue by adding to this complexity by stating that "the fact [is] that the interpreter-mediated health encounter reflects deep historical and contemporary sociopolitical, cultural, and economic divisions", specifically in the South African context due to our divisive past. Against this backdrop, language continues to play a central role in the lived experience, particularly of marginalisation, of fellow citizens. Furthermore, according to Benjamin et al. (2016: 74–75), the healthcare users who require interpreter services are very often not only among the most relegated in our society (i.e., socially, and economically), but also have a particularly painful past. As untrained interpreters frequently share the cultural and socioeconomic background of the patients, they may overidentify with the patient, and in the process be susceptible to fall victim to these dynamics and alliances within the interpreter-mediated encounter.

These are all problems that are aggravated in the context of mental healthcare, as diagnosis and consequent therapy of all conditions are heavily dependent on language use (Swartz et al. 2014). The key is taken from "[d]isordered language and communication [that] are commonly part of the symptomatology of serious mental disorder; where this is the case, the question of communication and interpretation is *not simply one of facilitating a discussion between two people* (clinician and healthcare user), each being able to communicate well, but in different languages" (Benjamin et al. 2016: 74–75; HML cursive).

Swartz et al. (2014: 2) also refer to some of the complexities of this in-between position of the interpreter:

> Interpreters may be erroneously assumed to be experts on the cultural and linguistic worlds of their clients and be asked to make complex judgements about the cultural acceptability of experiences service users may have. It is not uncommon for interpreters to be asked whether what would be regarded as hallucinations or delusions in western nosologies may in fact be culturally appropriate expressions of distress in the cultural world of health service users.

Apart from these challenges and shortcomings, the mere fact that the training of these ad hoc interpreters for mental healthcare could take place under the auspices of the Western Cape Health Department, and Department of Arts and Culture, in the form of a short course in collaboration with a tertiary institution is a step in the right direction. However, there is still room for improvement.

6 Discussion

What this paper signifies is that the relevant legislation for a multilingual language policy is in place as language policy played a seminal role in transforming the country from its divisive past. However, what one finds is that there are shortcomings and challenges when it comes to the implementation of the language policy in healthcare in Cape Town. To address these shortcomings on-site, ad hoc, or semi-skilled, including non-professional, interpreters are often used in healthcare. In a developing country with the division between a formal and informal economy, there is indeed room for these non(semi)-professionals, but the risks are high when it comes to service delivery and the lives of people.

These non(semi)-professionals also open the debate on interpreting quality as there often appears to be disparity between ideal (academic) quality and situated (real-world) quality. Although non(semi)-professionals do not live up to the academic norm, patients are generally appreciative to have someone who can facilitate the communication gap between themselves and the health professional when there is someone available who could speak on their behalf. From a (poor) real-world quality perspective, a descriptive approach should be adopted in healthcare interpreting. In such an approach we need to ask ourselves how a text *has been* interpreted and not how it *could be, could have been,* or *should have been* interpreted. This should also be the attitude in the case of healthcare interpreting, even though interpreters may deliver an interpreting service for the interim, and of which the academic quality is not up to scratch. Patients are still appreciative of the interpreter, irrespective of whether the interpreting service is non-professional.

Aside from the idealistic language-related and administration roles expected from semi-trained interpreters who are not equipped for the task at hand, with regard to mental health, the literature indicates that role-shifting (e.g., lay counsellors and administrators) is a reality. These unexpected effects including task-shifting were not foreseen, but if they persist, they could feed into curriculum development for the training of these interpreters.

Remote interpreting in the form of telephone interpreting is limited. On face value, however, it is a step in the right direction, but it also has its challenges, such as poor telephone connections, high costs, accents, and absence of non-verbal cues.

7 Conclusion

The absence and rather slow progress regarding the availability of professional language mediators in health services has led scholars to be skeptical about whether our healthcare system is serious about giving a voice to the non-English (i.e., indigenous SA language)-speaking patient. Certainly, within a developing context, there are various burning needs that compete for budget, but this should not discourage us in delivering a quality healthcare service.

The main finding of this paper is the confirmation that even though the legislative framework for a multilingual language policy for Cape Town is in place, the implementation of an efficient interpreting healthcare service is lacking. The tardiness in developing such a service to address the language impediments by instating professional language mediators in health services could lead one to doubt whether the healthcare system in the Cape metropole at least is indeed serious about giving fellow non-English-speaking patients a voice. Limited inroads have been made, as can be deduced from this paper, but further improvements are essential.

References

Antonini, R., L. Cirillo, L. Rossato, and I. Torresi. 2017. Introducing NPIT studies. In *Non-professional Interpreting and Translation: State of the art and future of an emerging field of research.* Amsterdam: John Benjamins Publishing Company.

Benjamin, E., L. Swartz, L. Hering, and B. Chiliza. 2016. Language barriers in health: Lessons from the experiences of trained interpreters working in public sector hospitals in the Western Cape. *South African Health Review* [Elcctronic], 2016(1). https://hdl.handle.net/10520/EJC189317. Accessed 4 Feb 2022.

Brink, E. 2014. An exploratory study on telephone interpreting in the Western Cape healthcare sector. Unpublished master's thesis. Stellenbosch: Stellenbosch University [Online].

Claassen, J., Z. Jama, N. Manga, M. Lewis, and D. Hellenberg. 2017. Building freeways: Piloting communication skills in additional languages to health service personnel in Cape Town. *South Africa. BMC Health Services Research* 17 (1): 390. https://doi.org/10.1186/s12913-017-2313-1.

Cole, P., L. Lawrence, N. Nyubuse, and J. Goddenet. 2003. *Costing the Western Cape Language Policy.* Cape Town: Emzantsi Associates.

Crawford, A. 1994. *Black Patients/White Doctors/Stories lost in Translation.* Cape Town: National Language Project.

Erasmus, M. ed. 1999. *Liaison interpreting in the community.* Pretoria: Van Schaik.

Feinauer, I., and H.M. Lesch. 2013. Health workers: Idealistic expectations versus interpreters' competence. *Perspectives: Studies in Translatology* 21(1):117–132. https://doi.org/10.1080/0907676X.2011.634013

Fine, D. 2001. Plain language communication: Approaches and challenges. In *Plain Legal language for Democracy*, eds. F. Viljoen and A. Nienaber, 17–26. Pretoria: Protea Bookhouse.

Hagan, S., X. Hunt, S. Kilian, B. Chiliza, and L. Swartz. 2020. Ad hoc interpreters in South African psychiatric services: Service provider perspectives. *Global Health Action* 13(1). https://doi.org/10.1080/16549716.2019.1684072

Karliner, L.S., E. Jacobs, A. Chen, and S. Mutha. 2007. Do professional interpreters improve clinical care for patients with limited English proficiency? A systematic review of the literature. *Health Services Research* 42 (2): 727–754. https://doi.org/10.1111/j.1475-6773.2006.00629.x.

Kelly, N. 2008. *Telephone interpreting: A comprehensive guide to the profession.* Lowell: Trafford.

Khumalo, T.R. 2015. Interpreting services provided during consultations in the medical sector: Identifying shortcomings. Unpublished master's thesis. Durban: Durban University of Technology.

Kilian, S., L. Swartz, and J. Joska. 2010. Competence of interpreters in a South African psychiatric hospital in translating key psychiatric terms. *Psychiatric Services* 61 (3): 309–312. https://doi.org/10.1176/ps.2010.61.3.309.

Leanza, Y. 2007. Role of community interpreters in pediatrics as seen by interpreters, physicians and researchers. In *Healthcare interpreting. Discourse and interaction*, eds. F. Pöchhacker and M. Shlesinger, 11–34. Amsterdam: Benjamins Publishing Company.

Lesch, H.M. 2007. Plain language for interpreting in consulting rooms. *Curationis* 30 (4): 73–78.

Lesch, H.M. 2009. *Interpreting Reader—A selection of essays.* Stellenbosch: Sunmedia.

Lesch, H.M. 2020. Investigating the effects of a (Non-)professional interpreting service in healthcare. *International Journal of Language and Linguistics* 7(4). https://doi.org/10.30845/ijll.v7n4p3

Lesch, H.M., and B. Saulse. 2014. Revisiting the interpreting service in the healthcare sector: A descriptive overview. *Perspectives: Studies in Translatology* [Electronic], 22 (3): 332–348. https://doi.org/10.1080/0907676X.2013.822008#.VHwfvDGUfV0

Levin, M. 2006. Language as a barrier to care for Xhosa-speaking patients at a South African paediatric teaching hospital. *South African Medical Journal* 96 (10): 1076–1079.

Maphumulo, W.T., and B.R. Bhengu. 2019. Challenges of quality improvement in the healthcare of South Africa post-apartheid: A critical review. *Curationis* 42 (1): e1–e9. https://doi.org/10.4102/curationis.v42i1.1901.

Monroe, A.D., and T. Shirazian. 2004. Challenging linguistic barriers to health care: Students as medical interpreters. *Academic Medicine* 79 (2): 118–122. https://doi.org/10.1097/00001888-200402000-00004.

Ndachi, M. 2014. Providing Health Care Interpreting in the Department of Radiation Oncology, Charlotte Maxeke Johannesburg Academic Hospital. Unpublished master's thesis. Johannesburg: University of the Witwatersrand.

Ntshona, M.S. 1999. Towards the development of an interpreting model for the health sector in South Africa. In *Liaison Interpreting in the community*, ed. M. Erasmus. Cape Town: Van Schaik.

Pfaff, C., and I. Couper. 2009. How do doctors learn the spoken language of their patients? *South African Medical Journal* [Electronic] 99(7): 520–522. https://www.ajol.info/index.php/samj/article/view/50798. Accessed 4 Feb 2022.

Saulse, B. 2010. Interpreting within the Western Cape Health Sector: A descriptive overview. Unpublished master's thesis. Stellenbosch: Stellenbosch University.

Schlemmer, A., and B. Mash. 2006. The effects of a language barrier in a South African District hospital. *Original Articles* 96 (10): 1080–1087.

Swartz, L., S. Kilian, J. Twesigye, D. Attah, and B. Chiliza. 2014. Language, culture and task shifting—An emerging challenge for global mental health. *Global Health Action* 7: 23433.

Van den Berg, V.L. 2016. Still lost in translation: Language barriers in South African health care remain. *South African Family Practice* 58 (6): 229–231. https://doi.org/10.1080/20786190.2016.1223795.

Williams, M., and S. Bekker. 2008. Language policy and speech practice in Cape Town: An exploratory public health sector study. *Southern African Linguistics and Applied Language Studies* 26 (1): 171–183. https://doi.org/10.2989/SALALS.2008.26.1.13.428

Wodak, R. 2013. What CDA is about—A summary of its history, important concepts and its developments. In *Methods of critical discourse analysis* [Electronic], eds. R. Wodak and M. Meyer, 1–13. SAGE. https://doi.org/10.4135/9780857028020.

Internet Sources

UN Migration. 2022a. *IOM South Africa* [Online]. https://southafrica.iom.int/publications/health-vulnerabilities-mobile-and-migrant-populations-and-around-port-durban-south-africa. Accessed 18 Oct 2021.

UN Migration. 2022b. *IOM South Africa* [Online]. https://southafrica.iom.int/. Accessed 18 Oct 2021.

Harold Lesch is associate professor at Stellenbosch University where he has established a training and research programme in interpreting. He originally qualified in translation studies and did research in this discipline. For the past 18 years he has been involved especially with interpreting training and interpreting research. He has produced a number of publications and papers on translation as well as interpreting, nationally and internationally. Furthermore, he has experience as a translator in the corporate sector, but also as a simultaneous interpreter in the national parliament of South Africa, the Western Cape Parliament and as a whisper interpreter. He also played a leading role in establishing an interpreting service on the campus of Stellenbosch University

Healthcare Interpreting Training: Present and Future at Spanish Universities

Almudena Nevado Llopis and Ana Isabel Foulquié-Rubio

1 Introduction

In Spain, there are 83 universities throughout its territory. Within this number, 50 are public universities and 33 are private universities (Secretaría General Técnica del Ministerio de Universidades 2021). In terms of the bachelor's degrees, the offer is very similar in most of them, even though the specialised modules in each degree may be slightly different from one university to the other. As for the master's degrees, each university designs its own and they are usually different from one university to the other, depending on its demand and priorities.

Regarding translation and interpretation degrees, they were firstly introduced in Spain at the end of the 1970s (Martin 2015: 3). From the onset, most bachelor's degrees included a high number of translation subjects and few interpreting subjects. Furthermore, and as explained by Martin (2015), interpreting subjects were mainly related to conference interpreting and other interpreting genres were not considered. Initially the curricula were more or less defined and analogous in all the degrees, therefore the subjects offered did not substantially differ from one university to another. Some decades later, with the implementation of the European Higher Education Area (EHEA), the countries involved agreed to and adopted various reforms in the universities based on common key values, such as self-government for institutions or academic freedom. In the case of Spain, through this process, the bachelor's degrees called *licenciaturas* (5-year degrees before the Bologna Process), which had

A. Nevado Llopis (✉)
Universidad San Jorge Campus Villanueva de Gállego, Autovía Zaragoza-Huesca km 510, 50830 Villanueva de Gállego, Zaragoza, Spain
e-mail: anevado@usj.es

A. I. Foulquié-Rubio
Universidad de Murcia, Murcia, Spain
e-mail: ana.foulquie@um.es

R. Lázaro Gutiérrez and C. Álvaro Aranda (eds.), *New Trends in Healthcare Interpreting Studies*, New Frontiers in Translation Studies,
https://doi.org/10.1007/978-981-99-2961-0_7

a more rigid structure and contents, were replaced by *grados* (4-year degrees after the Bologna Process), which allowed more flexibility and autonomy when designing their curricula. This modification entailed an opportunity to consider the social challenges and needs at that moment and, therefore, led to the inclusion of subjects related to public service interpreting or healthcare interpreting in the Spanish bachelor's degrees (Sales Salvador 2008; Martin 2015; Vargas Urpí 2016).

Precisely, the main aim of this chapter is to determine if translation and interpretation degrees are currently tailored to cover the needs regarding healthcare interpreting and to identify the characteristics that subjects and courses on this field should have.

In order to do so, the subjects dealing with healthcare interpreting offered by Spanish universities will be analysed in detail. It is important to clarify that only the subjects included in formal training, such as bachelor's degrees and official master's degrees, will be studied. Non-formal training in this field, usually provided by NGOs, private companies and associations (Álvaro Aranda and Gutiérrez 2021), will not be considered.

The collected data will provide a bigger picture of the current situation of healthcare interpreting training in Spain, describe its strengths and weaknesses and suggest measures for improvement in the future, in favour of the professionalisation of healthcare interpreting in this country.

This research is part of the work conducted within the framework of the Erasmus + Project ReACTMe.[1] The aim of the project was to provide healthcare interpreter training within universities to contribute to the professionalisation of healthcare interpreting. The means to this end were performing a comparative analysis of the current needs and potential responses regarding healthcare interpreting in Romania, Italy and Spain; providing tools for training healthcare interpreters; training trainers and higher education learners; and designing a curriculum for a joint blended learning module on healthcare interpreting to be implemented after the funding period at the participating higher education institutions.

2 Methodology

Our study used a mixed methodology, being the qualitative approach, in comparison with the quantitative approach, more relevant. Different data collection techniques were employed. On the one hand, a document analysis was conducted. Firstly, a search on different online tools was carried out in order to determine which Spanish universities offered translation and interpretation studies in the 2021–2022 academic year, both at undergraduate and postgraduate level. In particular, these tools were QUEDU (*Qué Estudiar y Dónde en la Universidad*) created by the Ministry of

[1] The acronym ReACTMe refers to Research & Action and Training in Medical Interpreting, an Erasmus + project focusing on healthcare interpreting in Spain, Italy and Romania involving six universities: San Jorge University, University of Murcia, University of Bologna, University of the International Studies of Rome, "Iuliu Hatieganu" University of Medicine and Pharmacy and Babeş-Bolyai University. For more information, visit http://reactme.net/home.

Education, Culture and Sport of the Spanish Government (https://www.educacion.gob.es/notasdecorte/busquedaSimple.action); Universia (https://www.universia.net/es/estudios), an open network which gathers more than 800 associated universities in 20 countries; and Educaweb (www.educaweb.com), a private educational website for academic and professional orientation.

As for the first tool, the search was refined by the type of degree (bachelor's or master's) and the keywords "translation",[2] "interpretation"[3] and "translation and interpretation" were used. Concerning the second tool, the search was refined by country (Spain), by the type of degree (bachelor's and master's degrees) and by knowledge area (being Arts and Humanities the area which corresponds to translation and interpretation studies). The same keywords used with the previous tool were employed with Universia and Educaweb. Double degrees including translation and interpretation were not considered in our study since they are usually combined with degrees such as philology, applied languages, foreign languages and literature, tourism or international relations, which are not related to healthcare, and their interpreting courses (if any) belong to the degree of translation and interpretation (Aguayo Arrabal 2019; Camacho Sánchez 2019).

The data obtained from these tools was contrasted and completed with the statistics shown in the document "TITULACIONES en universidades españolas. Curso 2020–2021" developed by the Spanish Register for Universities, Centres and Degrees (*Registro de Universidades, Centros y Titulaciones*, RUCT) and made available on the web page "Estadísticas e Informes Universitarios" of the Spanish Ministry of Education, as well as with the data provided in the report "Datos y cifras del Sistema Universitario Español. Publicación 2020–2021" developed by the General Technical Secretariat of the Spanish Ministry of Universities.

Once the Spanish universities offering translation and interpretation studies were detected, the curricula of these degrees were studied in search of interpreting subjects related to healthcare (i.e., Liaison and Consecutive Interpreting, Intercultural Mediation, Public Service Interpreting or specifically Healthcare Interpreting). Then the syllabi of those subjects were analysed to determine the following aspects: subject name, number of ECTS credits,[4] type of subject (compulsory, elective), year in which it is studied, language combination(s), methodology and learning outcomes (See Tables 1 and 2 in Sects. 4.1 and 4.2).

Additionally, with the aim of determining whether the languages offered in the interpreting subjects were appropriate to answer the needs of the linguistic and

[2] It is worth mentioning that, while most Spanish bachelor's degrees which only have "translation" in their name usually include in their curricula also interpreting subjects, this rule is not applied to all master's degrees only mentioning "translation" in their names, therefore in subsequent steps of the research process, the inclusion of interpreting subjects in these master's had to be verified.

[3] When using the keyword "interpretation" (*interpretación*) a careful verification had to be done, since this word may have different meanings in Spanish and, consequently, may refer to acting and musical performing.

[4] ECTS stands for the European Credit Transfer and Accumulation System. It was adopted by most of the countries in the European Higher Education Area as the national credit system and it allows credits taken at one higher education institution to be equally considered at another.

cultural minorities living in Spain, an analysis of the main migrant populations and the larger tourist communities was conducted through the Spanish Office for National Statistics (INE) website.

On the other hand, in December 2020 and January 2021, four focus groups with 25 participants in total were organised: two with healthcare interpreters working in both public and private Spanish hospitals; one with interpreting lecturers teaching in public and private universities distributed across the country; and one with heads of department and directors of translation and interpretation degrees. The focus groups were conducted online using videoconference tools (in particular, Microsoft Teams and Zoom). They were recorded and subsequently transcribed verbatim, anonymising the names of the participants by assigning them a code composed by a letter (I = interpreters; T = trainers; D = heads of department and directors) and a number depending on the order of intervention during the focus group. The issues discussed in these focus groups mainly dealt with the similarities and differences between the various interpreting settings (hospitals, courts, conferences, business settings, etc.), the role and the required competences for healthcare interpreters and their potential need for specialised training, and the most appropriate methods and resources to be used when training healthcare interpreters.

Finally, the data previously obtained was complemented with a literature review regarding translation and interpretation degrees, as well as public service and healthcare interpreting training.

3 Brief Description of the Spanish Demographical Context

Until the 1990s, Spanish migrants usually moved to France, Germany and South America to look for a better life. However, and probably due to its location and its entry in the European Union, among other factors, in the last 30 years, Spain has seen an appreciable rise in the number of immigrants. According to the latest available data provided by the Spanish National Institute of Statistics by the end of 2021, out of the 47,394,223 citizens residing in Spain, there are 5,434,153 foreign residents, 11.34% of the total population. Apart from the foreign residents, Spain has always been a very important tourist destination. Most of these tourists and immigrants, as will be detailed in the following paragraphs, come from countries where the official language is not Spanish. Consequently, in order to guarantee them quality care and equal rights when using our healthcare services, professional interpreting should be provided.

As for the numbers and origins, most immigrants come from European countries (2,179,998), America (1,554,087) and Africa (1,199,402). Regarding the specific countries, and considering only those whose mother tongue is not Spanish, the list is headed by Morocco (865,945), followed by Romania (667,378), the United Kingdom (262,885), Italy (252,008), China (232,807), Bulgaria (122,375), Ukraine (115,186), Germany (111,937), France (108,275), Brazil (98,655), Pakistan (97,705), Portugal

(97,628), Russia (82,788), Senegal (76,973), Algeria (66,893), India (54,387), Poland (53,418), the Netherlands (46,891) and the United States (40,712).

Concerning tourists, in 2019, before the pandemics, and according to the Spanish National Institute of Statistics, 83,701,011 visited Spain. The main countries of origin of these tourists were the United Kingdom (18,078,076), Germany (11,176,545) and France (11,156,671).

Evidently, not all these immigrants and tourists will need medical care, but according to previous studies which consider Spanish healthcare providers' experiences and opinions (Abril Martí and Martin 2011; Nevado Llopis 2015; Plaza Espuña et al. 2015; Román-López et al. 2015; Foulquié-Rubio and Beteta-Fernández 2020; Valero Garcés 2020), they usually find linguistic barriers when communicating with foreign patients and therefore we can conclude that there is a significant need for healthcare interpreting.

With these figures in mind, and before analysing the formal training in healthcare interpreting offered at Spanish universities, a brief description of the solutions given to these allophone patients should be conducted. In Spain, as in the other countries included in the ReACTMe project, translation and interpreting services provided in healthcare settings are not centrally organised but are mostly in the hands of regional bodies. Furthermore, the role of professional healthcare interpreters is not always recognised. Sometimes, in the best cases, language services are provided by cultural mediators and private companies employing anyone speaking a foreign language, but frequently lacking the professional knowledge and skills of a qualified interpreter. In many other cases, foreign patients have to rely on their own means to be able to communicate with healthcare professionals and they often have to resort to family members and other non-qualified ad hoc interpreters. This situation is sometimes derived from the lack of trained interpreters, especially with regard to languages of minor diffusion, but in other cases, the reason behind it is the lack of recognition and the idea that anyone who knows two languages is able to interpret. Unfortunately, in comparison, the situation concerning healthcare interpreting is not very different in other European countries. Even if the second decade of the twenty-first century has witnessed an increase in accreditation programs not only in the United States but also in other countries such as Australia, New Zealand, United Kingdom, Sweden, Switzerland, Ireland and Belgium (Tipton and Furmanek 2016: 116), there is still an absence of formal legislation and policy guidance concerning language access in health settings in the EU. Therefore, in many countries (such as Germany, Greece or Italy) professional interpreting services are rarely provided (Angelelli 2019: 36). An exception could be the United Kingdom, where legislation regulates the provision of interpreting for those patients who do not speak English, or the Netherlands, where professional interpreting services were consistently provided, but only until 2012, when they were cut out due to budget reductions (Zendedel et al. 2018: 158).

4 Healthcare Interpreting Training in Spain

At present, 31 out of the 83 Spanish universities mentioned in the introduction offer some kind of translation and interpretation training which is distributed in three levels: bachelor's degrees, master's degrees and doctoral studies.[5]

In terms of the data provided by the Spanish Register of Universities, Centres and Degrees and the online tools QEDU, Universia and Educaweb about translation and interpretation degrees, bachelor's degrees and official master's degrees will be analysed.

(a) Bachelor's Degrees:

In total, 31 Spanish universities offer a bachelor's degree in translation and interpretation (or some kind of variant, such as translation and intercultural communication, translation and linguistics or translation and intercultural mediation).

The curriculum of the translation and interpretation bachelor's degrees is very similar in most universities. In order to fulfil the requirements of the EHEA, students normally have to pass 240 ECTS in four years. Subjects such as Spanish (for students with Spanish as their mother tongue), Linguistics for Translators, Software and Editing Tools for Translators, among many others are usually offered in these bachelor's degrees. Students choose one B language (first foreign language) and one C language (second foreign language). Most universities offer English and French as B languages, but there are a few that include additional B languages, such as German or Arabic. The choice for C languages depends on the university, yet the most common are English and French, and less frequently German, Italian, Arabic, Russian, Chinese, etc. Then, students study a wide range of translation subjects from their B language and their C language. On the contrary, the quantity of compulsory subjects devoted to interpreting is usually kept to a minimum of 12–18 ECTS to which other elective interpreting subjects are sometimes added.

(b) Master's Degrees:

Master's degrees generally have a one-year duration and equate to 60 ECTS. There are 26 universities offering master's degrees in translation and/or interpretation in Spain. However, only 7 of them include the term interpretation in their name.

The master's degrees exclusively in translation are usually related to specialised fields of study, such as literary translation, legal translation, audiovisual translation, etc. Those focused on interpretation usually deal with conference interpreting. As an exception, there is a master's degree offered by the University of Alcalá which is devoted to public service interpreting and translation. Regarding master's degrees combining translation and interpretation, as in the case of the bachelor's degrees, most subjects are associated with translation and a very scarce number with interpreting.

[5] Doctoral studies will not be considered in this research, as they do not usually include subjects, which are the core element under study.

And now, with the main aim of this chapter in mind, the subjects similar or related to healthcare interpreting offered in these bachelor's and master's degrees will be analysed.

4.1 Healthcare Interpreting Subjects

Before delving into the analysis of the curricula, it should be mentioned that healthcare interpreting is normally included in subjects with a broader scope, such as Public Service Interpreting (which also deals with interpreting in other settings, as, for example, legal interpreting or police interpreting) and Intercultural Mediation, or even in more general interpreting subjects.[6] In fact, in the degrees under study there is only one subject which specifically includes healthcare interpreting in its name, which is offered by the University of Alcalá.

In total, there are 20 subjects that include healthcare interpreting training to some extent, offered at 12 universities.

If we classify the subjects according to the type of degree, 9 out of the 20 subjects are included in bachelor's degrees and 11 are included in master's degrees. It is important to highlight that this figure is based only on the contents, since, as we will see in the following section, the number of subjects increases if we take into account that, at the same university, different subjects with the same name may be offered depending on the language combination.

Table 1 below shows the provision for formal training in the field of healthcare interpreting:

Table 1 Subjects offered at Spanish universities with some content about healthcare interpreting

University	Degree	Name of the subject	ECTS	Type	Year
Autonomous University of Barcelona (UAB)	MA in Translation and Intercultural Studies	Introduction to Public Service Interpreting	5	E	
		Settings in Public Service Interpreting	5	E	
		Practices in Public Service Interpreting	5	E	

(continued)

[6] In some translation and interpretation degrees, healthcare interpreting is included in more general compulsory subjects, as the syllabus is usually left to the choice of the lecturer. An example of this would be the subject Introduction to Interpreting offered in the bachelor's degree in Translation and Interpretation at the University of Alicante.

Table 1 (continued)

University	Degree	Name of the subject	ECTS	Type	Year
Jaume I University (UJI)	BA in Translation and Interpretation	Intercultural Mediation and Interpretation A1—B/B—A1 in Public Service Domains	4.5	E	4
	MA in Medical and Healthcare Translation	Mediation in Healthcare Settings	4	E	
		Interpreting Techniques for Healthcare Settings	4	E	
	MA in Research in Translation and Interpretation	Methodology of Research in Intercultural Mediation and Translation in Healthcare Settings	5	E	
Pablo de Olavide University (UPO)	MA in International Communication, Translation and Interpreting	Social Interpreting	6	C	
San Jorge University (USJ)	BA in Translation and Intercultural Communication	Public Service Interpreting	6	E	4
		Intercultural Mediation	6	E	3
University of Alcalá (UAH)	MA in Intercultural Communication and Translation and Interpreting in Public Settings	Healthcare Interpreting	5	C	
University of Alicante (UA)	BA in Translation and Interpretation	Interpreting	6	C	3
University of Granada (UGR)	BA in Translation and Interpretation	Introduction to Public Service Interpreting B/C-A	6	E	4
University of Las Palmas de Gran Canaria (ULPGC)	MA in Professional Translation and Intercultural Mediation	Liaison Interpreting	6	E	
		Interpreting and Mediation in Public Services	6	E	
		Note-taking for Intercultural Mediation	6	E	
University of Murcia (UM)	BA in Translation and Interpretation	Public Service Interpreting B-A	6	C	4
University of Valladolid (UVa)	BA in Translation and Interpretation	Social Interpreting	3	E	4
University of Vic (UVic) and Open University of Catalonia (UOC)	BA in Translation, Interpretation and Applied Languages	Teleinterpretation	6	E	4
University of Vigo (UVIGO)	BA in Translation and Interpretation	Liaison Interpreting	6	E	3

E = elective; C = compulsory
The year in which the subjects are studied is only mentioned in the case of the bachelor's degrees, since all the master's degrees included in the table have a one-year duration

Concerning the type of subject, as explained in previous studies carried out by authors like Martin (2015), Camacho Sánchez (2019), and Álvaro Aranda and Lázaro Gutiérrez (2021),[7] Public Service Interpreting or related subjects are usually elective. There are very few exceptions, as for example the bachelor's degree in Translation and Interpretation offered by the UM, which after a modification of the curriculum in 2018, determined that the Public Service Interpreting subject would be compulsory for all the students in their B language, or the master's degree in International Communication, Translation and Interpreting offered by UPO, in which the Social Interpreting subject is also compulsory.

With regard to the course in which the subjects offered at an undergraduate level are studied, most of them are studied at the third or fourth year.

After this analysis of the Public Service Interpreting, Intercultural Mediation or related subjects at Spanish universities, the situation has not significantly changed in relation to the one depicted some years ago in some of the chapters of the monograph focused on public service translation and interpreting in Spain edited by Foulquié-Rubio et al. (2018) (see, for example, the chapters written by Nevado Llopis, for Aragón; Ugarte Ballester and Vargas Urpí, for Catalonia; Pérez-Luzardo Díaz and Fernández Pérez, for the Canary Islands; and Foulquié-Rubio, for Murcia).

4.2 Language Combinations

In this section we aim to determine if training related to healthcare interpreting offered by Spanish universities fulfils the language needs of interpreting in healthcare settings. In order to do so, we will consider the language combinations included in the translation and interpretation curricula and compare them with the data described in Sect. 3 about immigrants living in or tourists visiting Spain.

According to the foreign communities with a larger number of residents, the most demanded languages may be those spoken in Morocco,[8] Romanian, English, Italian and the languages spoken in China.[9] To a lesser extent, other demanded languages may be Bulgarian, Ukrainian, German and French. As for tourists, English, French and German are likely to be the languages with greater demand. The distribution of immigrants and tourists is not homogeneous among the different Spanish regions.

[7] Our findings differ to some extent from the study presented by Camacho Sánchez (2019), as we have included only those subjects specifically mentioning healthcare interpreting training in their syllabi, and from the study conducted by Álvaro Aranda and Gutiérrez (2021), as it was mainly based on the data obtained through interviews with the lecturers of the different subjects under study.

[8] Morocco is a multilingual country. The two official languages are Standard Arabic and Tamazight, while Moroccan Arabic (known as Darija) is the spoken native vernacular.

[9] The main language in China is Standard Chinese, which is based on central Mandarin, but there are hundreds of related Chinese languages which differ from each other both morphologically and phonetically.

Concerning the language combinations offered at the bachelor's and master's degrees including subjects related to healthcare interpreting, Table 2 below provides information on their B, C or D languages:

Table 2 Languages offered in translation and interpretation degrees in Spain

University	Degree	B language/s	C language/s	D language/s
Autonomous University of Barcelona (UAB)	MA in Translation and Intercultural Studies	Chinese English		
Jaume I University (UJI)	BA in Translation and Interpretation	English	German French	
	MA in Medical and Healthcare Translation	English		
	MA in Research in Translation and Interpretation	English		
Pablo de Olavide University (UPO)	MA in Research in Translation and Interpretation	English		
San Jorge University (USJ)	BA in Translation and Intercultural Communication	English	French	
University of Alcalá (UAH)	MA in Intercultural Communication and Translation and Interpreting in Public Settings	Arabic Chinese English French Russian		
University of Alicante (UA)	BA in Translation and Interpretation	English French German	English French German	Arabic Chinese Italian Polish Romanian Russian Greek
University of Granada (UGR)	BA in Translation and Interpretation	Arabic English French German	Arabic Chinese English French German Greek Italian Portuguese Russian	
University of Las Palmas de Gran Canaria (ULPGC)	MA in Professional Translation and Intercultural Mediation	English		

(continued)

Table 2 (continued)

University	Degree	B language/s	C language/s	D language/s
University of Murcia (UM)	BA in Translation and Interpretation	English French	Arabic English French German Italian	
University of Valladolid (UVa)	BA in Translation and Interpretation	English	French German	
University of Vic (UVic) and Open University of Catalonia (UOC)	BA in Translation, Interpretation and Applied Languages	English	French German	
University of Vigo (UVIGO)	BA in Translation and Interpretation	English French	English French German Portuguese	

At an undergraduate level, the language combinations offered by most bachelor's degrees in translation and interpretation is Spanish as an A language (mother tongue)[10] and English as a B language. Some bachelor's degrees offer French as a B language, and the number of degrees offering German as a B language is very small. UGR is the only university that offers Arabic as a B language. The most common C languages offered in the bachelor's degrees under study are Italian, French and Arabic, but there are universities that offer the chance to also study German or Russian as C languages (in particular, UGR and UAB). Finally, some bachelor's degrees offer the possibility to also study a D language, as for example UA, which includes Polish, Romanian and Russian[11] as D languages. This D language is taught as an additional language, but there are no interpreting subjects related to it. As for the specific subjects analysed in the previous section, most of them are only taught in the B language (English, French, German and Arabic), and only the subject offered by UGR includes the C language. This is usually the rule with all the interpreting subjects, not only the ones dealing with public service and healthcare interpreting, since it is assumed that there is not enough time for students to master their C language to a level that would allow them to interpret.

At a postgraduate level, there is only one master's degree that includes different language combinations. This is the case of the master's offered by UAH which, according to the information published on its website, has different combinations including Arabic, Chinese, French, English and Russian.

---

[10] An exception would be the universities in the regions in which there are other official languages, such as Catalan, Galician or Basque that are usually also included as an A language.

[11] It is worth mentioning that the wide range of languages in the UA curriculum is something exceptional, as most curricula include only B and C languages, and the range is usually the same.

Observing the objective data (language combinations offered and migrant and tourist populations), the training provided in Spanish bachelor's and master's degrees in translation and interpretation, at first sight, does not fulfil the needs of healthcare interpreting services. This was corroborated somehow by the participants in the focus groups who justify the exclusion of languages of minor diffusion by the scarce number of students normally enrolled in subjects with these language combinations and the consequent scarce economic profitability of them. Nevertheless, they consider that students whose mother tongue is foreign and not included in the curricula may apply their acquired interpreting knowledge and skills to that language in the future. In particular, one of the trainers explains:

> Y podría ofrecerse mucho más. Por ejemplo, yo sé que hay un máster también de estudios árabes y sería interesante que esa combinación se añadiera en los estudios de interpretación, y otras muchísimas lenguas de la realidad de aquí de España y de nuestra ciudad en concreto. Que luego, evidentemente tenemos alumnos de origen extranjero, con lengua materna, por ejemplo, árabe o chino, y una vez adquirida la técnica podrán hacerlo con su idioma, pero no se ofrece en las combinaciones que reflejarían mejor la situación de aquí. [And offering much more would be possible. For example, I know there is a master's degree on Arabic studies and adding this combination to interpretation studies would be interesting, as well as many other languages in line with the Spanish reality and specifically with the reality of our city. Evidently, we have many foreign students whose mother tongue is, for example, Arabic or Chinese, and once they have acquired the technique, they will be able to apply it to their language, but we do not offer the language combinations which would better reflect our reality.] (T4)

Additionally, when talking about languages of minor diffusion, it should be highlighted that dialectal varieties have to be considered, especially in the case of Arabic, and mainly due to the fact that the origin of the highest number of foreign residents in Spain is Morocco. One of the trainers agrees with this idea and argues:

> Quería además añadir que el hecho de tener árabe en la carrera de traducción e interpretación como lengua C no es una garantía de que sea el árabe que van a utilizar cuando interpreten, porque ellos estudian el árabe clásico y en servicios públicos se necesita más el Dariya. [I would like to add that offering Arabic as a C language in the translation and interpretation degrees does not guarantee that this will be the language used when interpreting, because classic Arabic is studied in the degree, while in public services, Dariya (the Moroccan variety) is more needed.] (T1)

As previously stated, the language combination mostly taught is English–Spanish-English and to a lesser extent other B languages, such as French, German and Arabic. On the one hand, according to some participants in the focus groups, it is adequate to teach public service interpreting in the combination English–Spanish-English, as English is widely used as lingua franca in healthcare settings. On the other hand, according to some participants, offering only English as a B language is not enough, as stated by one trainer who expounds:

> Aquí sí que hay una demanda enorme de interpretación. Y nosotros en los grados solo ofrecemos como lengua B inglés, porque con el paso de las licenciaturas a los grados se aprovechó para meterle un buen tijeretazo a las titulaciones y reducir la oferta. Y se pasó de tener las lenguas B francés, alemán e inglés, a solo ofrecer inglés como lengua B y, entonces, tenemos las lenguas C francés y alemán exclusivamente. Por tanto, antes se llegaba a un nivel

de profundidad en el estudio de la lengua que no se llega hoy en día ni con el alemán, que es muy preocupante, ni con el francés, que es más preocupante todavía. Y ya empezamos a ver las consecuencias de eso, porque resulta muy difícil en nuestra comunidad encontrar a alguien que esté bien preparado con un fuerte alemán, o un fuerte francés para hacer frente a la gran demanda que hay. [Here there is a strong demand for interpreting. In our bachelor's degrees we only offer English as a B language because the change from *licenciaturas* to *grados* was used to snip the degrees and reduce what was offered. Therefore, before we had French, German and English as B languages, but now we have only English as a B language and French and German exclusively as C languages. Consequently, the high level of German and French that was acquired at that time is not reached nowadays, which is very worrying. Now we are witnessing the consequences of this, because it is really difficult in our region to find someone who is fluent in German or French in order to meet the high demand.] (T5)

In short, most universities do not consider the migrant and tourist populations when designing the curriculum of translation and interpretation degrees and, therefore, the language combinations offered in the subjects under study do not fulfil the needs of interpreting in the Spanish healthcare services.

4.3 Role and Required Competences for Healthcare Interpreters

Concerning the professional role, according to the interpreters participating in the focus groups, there are many differences between a healthcare interpreter and, for example, a legal or a conference interpreter. This is mainly caused by the healthcare interpreters' relation with both parties, their physical contact with the patient, the emotional implication and the importance of nonverbal language (gestures, tone of voice, facial expressions, etc.). They consider that healthcare interpreters perform many tasks that other interpreters working in different settings would not perform; for example, in their opinion, healthcare interpreters try to create an initial climate of trust; sometimes they have to calm the patient down; they frequently double-check if the patient has understood everything; occasionally, they speak with the patient and their relatives before entering the consultation room and ask them the customary questions in advance to save time (as time is essential in healthcare settings), etc. In their view, some of these tasks are related to the fact that one of the parties involved (the patient) is in a disadvantaged position, as they usually do not have any kind of knowledge about how the healthcare system works and its different procedures, and that causes greater empathy towards them.

The asymmetrical relation between the parties (the healthcare professional and the foreign-speaking patient) is also pointed out by the directors and heads of department participating in the focus group, as this director clearly depicts:

Lo que los diferencia es la situación de la comunicación. Un intérprete de conferencias es un intérprete canal, es decir, él no interviene en el intercambio comunicativo más que como canal que vehicula el mensaje. Sin embargo, un intérprete sanitario lo que hace es que facilita la comunicación, en el sentido de que ecualiza los términos de la ecuación. Un intérprete de conferencias tiene usuarios que tienen unos conocimientos y un rango muy

> parecidos, simplemente no hablan el mismo idioma. En el caso de un intérprete sanitario, los usuarios son muy distintos por su formación. Tenemos un médico, y tenemos un paciente que no sabemos ni siquiera qué tipo de formación tiene, ni si comprende el idioma, ni siquiera si se le está interpretando hacia su lengua materna. Entonces, ahí el intérprete lo que hace es que abre y cierra la puerta de la comunicación, pide explicaciones a las diferentes personas para poder transmitir mejor el mensaje, porque no se está entendiendo adecuadamente. El intérprete sanitario es como el guardián de la puerta, por así decirlo, que crea un triángulo comunicativo. [What differentiates them is the communicative situation. A conference interpreter is a channel, I mean, they only intervene in the communicative exchange as a channel that conveys the message. On the contrary, a healthcare interpreter facilitates communication, in the sense that they equalise the terms of the equation. Users of conference interpreting have very similar knowledge and status; they simply do not speak the same language. The users of healthcare interpreting are very different regarding their training. There is a doctor and there is a patient whose training is unknown, and we do not know if the patient understands the language or even if we are interpreting into their mother tongue. Therefore, here the interpreter opens and closes the communication door, asks for clarifications to the different parties in order to be able to correctly convey the message, because it is not being properly understood. The healthcare interpreter is like the guardian of the door, in other words, who creates a communicative triangle.] (D2)

In that regard, the directors and heads of department believe that healthcare interpreters act as linguistic and cultural mediators, in the sense that they have to understand the language and the culture and adapt their message to that specific culture, sometimes giving explanations. This idea is also supported by some of the interpreters. Regarding this issue, one of them explains:

> Creo que el componente de identificación y de empatía con el paciente es fundamental, pero también teniendo mucho en cuenta que es un elemento que creo que se debe destacar en la formación. Porque el intérprete, aunque a veces actúe como mediador, debe estar formado para ponerse a sí mismo unos límites y no forzar a los pacientes a que vayan más allá de lo que querrían decir, al tiempo que además va a tener que ver si los pacientes se están quedando cortos con respecto a la información que se les pide, pues por elementos culturales, por timidez… Y además debe ser capaz de detectar si el médico no está aportando suficiente información o el canal que ha elegido no es el adecuado, y comprobará que el paciente responda a lo que realmente el médico quiere saber. Entonces, creo que el aspecto formativo en ese sentido es primordial. [I think that the component of identification and empathy towards the patient is basic, but this is a fact that should be highlighted during the training. Because interpreters, although they sometimes act as mediators, they should be trained to limit themselves and not force the patients to go beyond what they want to say. And at the same time, the interpreter should see if the patients are falling short in relation with what has been requested, due to cultural elements, because they are shy… And besides, the interpreter should be able to detect if the doctor is not giving enough information or has chosen an inadequate channel and should check if the patient is answering the doctor's questions. In conclusion, I believe that training is fundamental in that sense.] (I12)

At this point, it is worth mentioning that the coexistence of the two profiles, intercultural mediators and interpreters, has been present in Spain for the last decades, sometimes even exchanging their roles and functions. The discussion goes beyond the scope of this chapter, but we agree with Vargas Urpí (2016), who states that this coexistence has made the distinction between the two profiles difficult and it may even have hindered the professionalisation of public service interpreting.

Additionally, the heads of department and the trainers think that all kinds of interpreters share the basic techniques and competences, but there are differences, for example, concerning terminology or the context in which they work and its protocols, and especially, as in the case of the interpreters participating in the focus groups, they highlight the importance of the emotional implication and the necessary management of emotions in healthcare settings. Moreover, the trainers point out the turn-taking management as a difference between court/legal interpreting (where the conversation is more hierarchical and rigid) and healthcare interpreting (where the short physical distance and the type of conversation allow the interpreter, for example, to ask questions if needed).

Another important differentiating factor mentioned by some interpreters is the unpredictability and immediacy of most of their interventions and the consequent lack of previous specific preparation (as opposed, for example, to conference interpreters). In relation to this immediacy, both the interpreters and the trainers talk about the unexpected situations that may happen in healthcare settings and the need to make decisions on short notice.

Furthermore, the dramatic consequences that an error made by a healthcare interpreter (or a court interpreter) may have (unlike the consequences of an error in, for example, conference interpreting) are mentioned by the participants in the four focus groups.

Finally, the interpreters report the lack of recognition of healthcare interpreters in comparison to conference interpreters (issue that is noted on many occasions during the focus groups with interpreters). In the words of one of the interpreters:

> A lo mejor el intérprete de conferencias está más... es más conocida la figura y está más reconocida. Y a lo mejor el intérprete de servicios públicos o el intérprete sanitario está todavía a caballo un poco entre la profesionalización y la invasión o el intrusismo laboral. [Perhaps conference interpreters are more known and more recognised. And perhaps public service interpreters or healthcare interpreters are still halfway in between the professionalisation and the invasion or the unauthorised practice of the profession.] (I8)

As a consequence of the differences observed by them, all the participants in the focus groups consider there should be some specific training for healthcare interpreters. In this respect, an interpreter maintains the idea that training is a necessary step for healthcare interpreters' professionalisation and points out:

> Yo creo que la formación es esencial si queremos profesionalizarnos. O sea, para que nuestro trabajo se considere una profesión, no una ocupación como ocurre de momento... Entonces, para que nosotros pasemos a ser una profesión regularizada, pues la formación es absolutamente esencial, porque una educación, por ejemplo, universitaria, ayudaría al reconocimiento de la profesión. Habría un control social y habría una acreditación... En resumidas cuentas, nos ayudaría mucho que se dedicaran a este trabajo personas bien formadas, sea cual sea el tipo de formación, y profesionales. [I believe that training is essential if we want to become professionals. I mean, to make people consider our job as a profession, not as an occupation as it is considered at the moment. Therefore, to become a regulated profession, training is absolutely essential, since education, for example, at a university level, would stimulate the recognition of this profession. There would be a social control and an accreditation... In short, it would be very helpful that well trained people, regardless of the type of training they have received, would work in this setting.] (I5)

Concerning healthcare interpreters' training, most heads of department and directors believe that it should be very specialised and offered in a master's degree or a postgraduate course, which coincides with the idea disseminated after the implementation of the EHEA which suggests having bachelor's degrees which are generalist, and only include specialised courses in their final years. This suggestion is not totally applied in practice, since, as we have seen in Sect. 4.1, almost half of the subjects under analysis are taught at an undergraduate level, although they are generally studied in the third and fourth year of the bachelor's degrees. In that regard, and talking specifically about the interpreting subjects offered at Spanish universities, Martin (2015: 93) maintains that:

> España, por tanto, empezó una formación en interpretación de conferencia que iba en contra de la experiencia acumulada de otros países. Por esta razón, consideramos que la Licenciatura nació potencialmente viciada de raíz en cuanto a su componente troncal de interpretación. Quizás uno de los principales errores del plan de estudios de la Licenciatura fue el considerar la interpretación de conferencia como el único género de interpretación existente, lo cual llevó a la inclusión de las técnicas de interpretación más usadas en ese género. Sin embargo, existen otros géneros de interpretación, tales como la interpretación de acompañamiento, la interpretación social/en servicios públicos, la interpretación para el comercio y el turismo, que no están asociados a las técnicas de consecutiva y simultánea, y sí a la técnica de interpretación de enlace, por ejemplo, más asequible para los estudiantes, máxime teniendo en cuenta el número limitado de horas y las carencias en competencias instrumentales de muchos estudiantes de pregrado. [Therefore, Spain implemented conference interpreting training that went against the experience amassed by other countries. For this reason, we consider that the *licenciatura* was born potentially corrupted regarding the compulsory status of interpreting. Perhaps one of the main errors of the curriculum of this degree was considering conference interpreting as the unique interpreting genre which led to the inclusion of the techniques most frequently used in this genre. Nevertheless, there are other interpreting genres, as escort interpreting, social/public service interpreting, or interpreting in business and tourism settings, which are not associated to consecutive and simultaneous techniques, but to liaison interpreting techniques, for example, that are more feasible for students, especially considering the limited number of hours and the limitations concerning instrumental competencies of many undergraduate students.]

Along the same lines, one of the heads of department elucidates:

> ANECA publicó en 2004 un Libro Blanco sobre el Grado en Traducción e Interpretación, que dice básicamente que la interpretación debe ser un ámbito relevante, que no hay que renunciar a ella porque está incluido en la propia denominación del título. El planteamiento inicial era básicamente incluir una introducción a la interpretación y simplemente que se hiciera interpretación enlace, que no hubiera ni interpretación simultánea ni interpretación consecutiva. Pero se llegó al acuerdo de que se podía ir un poquito más allá de esos límites […] Y el Libro Blanco habla en varias ocasiones de la interpretación social, no habla para nada de interpretación en servicios públicos. Es un palabro que no existe en el Libro Blanco. Entonces, sí que tendría cabida, no como asignatura, pero sí como un tema de una asignatura, pues la interpretación sanitaria. Al final, tenemos 240 créditos a nuestra disposición, cuatro años, y hay que hacer encajes para cómo colocamos todo, y pasa lo que siempre pasa con la manta, es decir, o me tapo la cabeza o me tapo los pies, pero todo el cuerpo no me lo voy a poder tapar porque son muy pocos créditos para una formación tan compleja. [In 2004, ANECA, the Spanish National Agency for Quality Evaluation and Accreditation, published a document called White Paper about the bachelor's degree in translation and interpretation, and this document states that interpreting is a relevant field that cannot be eliminated, since

> it is included in the name of the degree. The initial plan was to include an introduction to interpreting and simply doing liaison interpreting, not including simultaneous or consecutive interpreting. But then, there was an agreement according to which there was the opportunity to go beyond those limits [...]. And the White Paper refers to, on many occasions, social interpreting. It does not mention public service interpreting, since it is a mouthful that does not exist within the White Paper. So, healthcare interpreting may have a place, not as a subject, but as a unit of a subject. Ultimately, we have 240 credits in 4 years at our disposal and we should juggle to fit everything in. It is always the same as with a blanket: I can cover my head or cover my feet, but I cannot cover my full body, as there are not enough credits for such complex training.] (D4)

On the other hand, the interpreters think that this training should not necessarily be provided in a full university degree. In their opinion, it could be a shorter non-formal course/module. This idea is also supported by authors such as Burdeus-Domingo et al. (2021) or Vargas Urpí (2016: 100), who explains that this kind of courses usually entail a win–win situation both for students and trainers as students receive tools and resources to facilitate their daily job and trainers get information and feedback about real professional situations.

Although it is true that this kind of non-formal courses are usually based on pragmatic and, in a certain way, intuitive criteria, since their main aim is answering the needs of the training developers, their basic contents are not so far from those included in formal training (Abril Martí and Martin 2008: 112).

With regard to the knowledge, skills and attitudes that healthcare interpreters should develop, for most interpreters participating in the focus groups, empathy is fundamental, but at the same time, it is essential to know how to deal with the emotional impact, to keep a distance from the lived situations, not to become too involved in them and, therefore, to avoid stress and trauma. In this sense, resilience/endurance is considered the cornerstone of the healthcare interpreter's work. Some interpreters state that they miss some psychological preparation to face the usual difficult situations they live. One of them, in particular, explains:

> Sí he tenido alguna defunción, sí he tenido que dar algunas noticias malas, sí he tenido algún paciente que va... muy malito y te escribe a las dos, tres semanas la familia diciendo "Muchas gracias, pero llegó muy mal". Hay momentos difíciles y es verdad que se agradecería muchísimo un apoyo, apoyo psicológico. Tampoco voy a decir constante, pero sí tener dónde recurrir y cómo... aprender a gestionar estas cosas. Porque... también es verdad que yo al principio me llevaba todo a casa [...] era muy sentida. Luego tiendes a relativizar un poco a coña... Desarrollas un cierto humor, no sé si negro o grisáceo oscuro, pero sí que... sí que ayuda, ayuda a enfrentarte a eso. Pero esas herramientas, en lugar de tener que desarrollarlas tú y a veces estrellarte contra ellas, pues sería de agradecer que las dieran antes. [I have had some deaths, I have had to give bad news, I have had some patients that arrived at the hospital in bad conditions and, after two or three weeks, the family wrote me saying "Thank you, but he/she was very ill". There are difficult moments and I would really be grateful if there were some support, psychological support, not necessarily constant, but to know where to turn to and how to do it... learn how to manage these situations. Because... it is true that at the beginning I used to take on everything [...] I was very sensitive. Afterwards we tend to minimise and somehow joke about it... We develop a kind of black humour, I do not know if it is black or greyish, but it does... it does help to face this. But these tools, instead of having to develop them by yourself and sometimes come across them, I would have really appreciated if I had received them beforehand.] (I2)

The heads of department also highlight the importance of being empathic (and respectful) and at the same time being able to deal with complicated and emotionally charged situations, showing psychological fortitude. In that respect, like the interpreters, they consider that teaching strategies to cope with these situations should be included in training.

When the need for these competences is searched in the learning outcomes section of the Spanish interpreting subjects, empathy is only found once, and resilience/endurance or psychological fortitude are hardly ever mentioned; the nearest concept (included in the syllabus of some subjects) is stress management. In this respect, it should be taken into account that some analysed subjects are related to interpreting (in general terms) instead of being focused on public service interpreting, healthcare interpreting, (intercultural) mediation or similar areas.

Additionally, in the interpreters' opinion, it is necessary to know how the hospital or clinic works, as well as the different procedures and documents used in these contexts. On that issue, the heads of department add the knowledge of the foreign-speaking patients' healthcare system. The trainers state that knowing the structure of the consultation, the basics of the medical interview, history-taking and diagnosis in different contexts (emergency, primary care, medical specialities) would also help. Considering that there is a very small quantity of subjects specifically focused on healthcare interpreting, the presence of this contextual and communicative knowledge in the learning outcomes section is very scarce (only two or three subjects specifically note it and some simply cite the more general thematic knowledge).

Moreover, the participants in the four focus groups mention the knowledge of the working languages and the related cultures (what is also included in the syllabus of the vast majority of subjects). Many issues arise about these two topics.

Concerning languages, there is one interpreter, one trainer and one head of department who stress the importance of knowing not only the standard language, but also the dialects and varieties spoken by the most usual patients. As for the subjects, the knowledge of different dialects, varieties and registers regarding the two working languages is included in many analysed syllabi.

In relation to cultures, the heads of department and directors and the trainers emphasise the importance of knowing the healthcare culture of the two parties involved. Furthermore, according to the interpreters, it is important to be aware of aspects such as religious beliefs (i.e., Jehovah Witnesses and their refusal of blood transfusions), taboo topics (i.e., menstruation) or traditions (i.e., burial habits) and be modest and ask if there is lack of such knowledge. On that subject, an interpreter explains:

> Como intérprete, tienes que saber de la cultura. No solamente… pues, por ejemplo, que en Holanda o en Inglaterra entierran a los diez días y no a las 24 horas, como en España. Entonces, cuando aquí se llevan al fallecido, los familiares, no tienen ni idea de lo que va a pasar. Son cosas que parecen muy sencillas y no son nada de traducir, pero si no las sabes puedes meter la gamba hasta el fondo y hacer mucho daño, tanto en la interpretación, como en lo personal hacia los pacientes y su familia. [As an interpreter, you should have cultural knowledge. Not only… for example, that in the Netherlands or in England people are buried after 10 days and not after 24 hours like in Spain. And therefore, when the deceased is taken, the relatives do not know what is going to happen. These are things that seem very simple,

that are not related to translation, but if you do not know them, you can make a big mistake and do harm, not only regarding interpreting, but also personally towards the patients and their families.] (I1)

Having cultural knowledge of the two communities involved is mentioned in many learning outcomes sections of the subjects under analysis, but only two subjects include healthcare culture knowledge as well. In addition, the intercultural mediation and some interpreting subjects refer to the ability to work in multicultural contexts.

On the other hand, the prerequisite of not being an apprehensive or impressionable person is also noted by the heads of department and directors. They, together with the trainers, additionally stress the need of knowing interpreting techniques, something that surprisingly is not mentioned by the interpreters. Regarding the interpreting techniques, practising liaison interpreting and bidirectionality is emphasised by the trainers. All the interpreting subjects cite interpreting techniques (some of them in general and others specifically —consecutive & note-taking, liaison, simultaneous, sight translation– depending on the nature of the subject). Within the interpreting techniques, the remote modes (telephone or videoconference interpreting) are not specifically mentioned by the participants in the focus groups, when these are modes more and more frequently used in recent years. In this respect, only a few studied degrees, such as the joint bachelor's degree offered by UVic and UOC, include subjects on liaison interpreting by telephone and videoconference. In terms of interpreting techniques, some general abilities and skills are also mentioned in some syllabi, such as memory, concentration, analysis and synthesis, mental agility, public speaking, etc., that, according to Martin (2015: 91), are not only in line with the interpretative theory of translation of Seleskovitch and Lederer (which, even if dated back to the 1960s, is still valid), but are also recommended by more recent accredited authors, such as Nolan (2005) and Gillies (2004, 2013).

Other general competences that appear in the learning outcomes section of some subjects are ability to reflect, critical thinking, self-analysis, ability to identify and solve problems, ability to make decisions, and ability to work autonomously and in teams.

Unpredictably, ethics is not specifically mentioned by any of the participants in the focus groups when talking about competences (although this issue is mentioned when talking about methods, as we will see in the following section), and only 10% of the subjects (approx.) specifically refer to the knowledge of professional deontology and ethics and some of the main ethical principles (especially, faithfulness and confidentiality).

Finally, interpersonal competence is also pointed out by the interpreters and the trainers as well as in the syllabus of a few subjects: turn-taking management, the ability to make the parties understand the interpreter's role, the capacity to negotiate and debate, assertiveness, etc. On this subject, one of the trainers explains:

Es de lo que más me confirman los estudiantes que acaban trabajando en el sector médico es esa necesidad de ser flexible, deben aprender a flexibilizar y a negociar. Primero, porque las cosas no están tan protocolizadas como están en otros sectores, como el judicial y el policial. Y segundo, porque la posibilidad de eventualidades y sorpresa se multiplica por dos, tres, cuatro o más si quieres, e incluso la manera de llevar a cabo la interacción la puedes estar negociando tres veces en una misma mañana. [One of the aspects mostly confirmed by the students who become medical interpreters is the need to be flexible; they must learn to be flexible and negotiate. Firstly, because things are not as much protocolised as they are in other settings, such as the courts or the police settings. Secondly because the chance of eventualities and surprise is multiplied by two, three, four, or more... and even the way in which interaction takes place may be negotiated three times during the same morning.] (T6)

4.4 Methods and Resources to Train Healthcare Interpreters

Concerning the resources and materials used for teaching/learning healthcare interpreting, the first and most appreciated resource mentioned by the trainers participating in the focus group is Linkterpreting (http://linkterpreting.uvigo.es/), an open access platform developed by Del Pozo Triviño, a lecturer and researcher at UVIGO, containing audio recorded role-plays (English–Spanish) to practise liaison interpreting and also including some preparatory exercises (paraphrasing and simplification, definitions, improvisation, etc.). In addition, they remark the mock exams provided by the certification bodies of the United States (i.e., Certification Commission for Healthcare Interpreters) or the United Kingdom (Institute of Linguists). They also highlight the materials developed by Cross-Cultural Communications, such as InterpreTIPS (https://www.youtube.com/channel/UCNjL_WcM4BIBw1L0X_ls63Q/featured), but, according to them, the problem with these materials is that they are linguistically and culturally distant from the Spanish reality, as shown in these trainers' words:

> Yo a veces recurro a los recursos del contexto estadounidense. Y siempre les digo a los alumnos en un mundo ideal tendríamos estos recursos aquí también. [I sometimes use resources which have been created in the USA. And I always tell my students that in an ideal world we would have this kind of resources here too.] (T5)

> Sí, yo me he comprado, por ejemplo, todos los materiales que ha ido sacando Marjory Bancroft,[12] que están muy bien, pero yo encuentro que los roles están tan alejados culturalmente y la lengua... que no puedo, no puedo justificar la utilización continuada de estos materiales en clase porque no tiene nada que ver con lo que nosotros estamos intentando hacer aquí, que es formar a personas que normalmente van a trabajar aquí. [Yes, I have bought, for example, all the materials developed by Marjory Bancroft, which are great, but I believe that the roles are culturally and linguistically far away... so I cannot justify the continuous use of these materials in class, since they are not related at all with what we are trying to do here, that is training people who will likely work here.] (T1)

As for medical terminology, the trainers explain that it is mainly taught through drawings and videos. All in all, in general, they all agree that there is a lack of teaching materials and resources to practise interpreting in healthcare settings.

With regard to the studied subjects during the document analysis stage, no specific resources are mentioned in the methodology section of their open access syllabi, with the exemption of some interpreting subjects which cite the use of speeches

[12] Marjory Bancroft was founder and director of Cross-Cultural Communications, a national training agency for medical and community interpreting operating in the USA.

from the European Commission webpage, recordings of the plenary sessions of the European Parliament, programmes of the Europe by Satellite Channel and the platform Interpreter Training Resources (https://interpretertrainingresources.eu/).

In relation to the methods, from the methodology section of the subjects, it can be inferred that they are mainly practical and little space is devoted to theory (only some master classes and readings about the different interpreting modes, the role of the interpreter and the profession, etc.).

In general, cooperative and problem-solving learning are preferred, and debates and teamwork are emphasised. Regarding the practical exercises mentioned in the methodology section of the analysed syllabi, they could be divided in pre-interpreting exercises (analysis and synthesis, memory, rephrasing, thematic research, and glossary development, etc.) and interpreting exercises (associated with different techniques: simultaneous, consecutive and note-taking, liaison, sight translation). In relation to the problem-solving techniques, which are also very useful in healthcare interpreting training, according to a study conducted by Álvaro Aranda and Gutiérrez (2021), these are generally included in the Public Service Interpreting subjects offered at Spanish universities; among them, clarification requests, the use of synonyms or the reformulation and self-correction strategies are highlighted in the aforementioned study.

Broadly speaking, role-plays are valued as an adequate method both in the analysed subjects and by the trainers. According to the information provided in some methodology sections of the studied syllabi, some role-plays are recorded and afterwards watched to examine the interpreting students' strengths and weaknesses and to make them learn from the mistakes made. In the trainers' view, the problem is that, if you cannot count on two lecturers and the students have to do the role of the parties themselves, they find it difficult to improvise. In this respect, the trainers consider that involving healthcare professionals in simulations and practising with non-scripted role-plays would be ideal. This suggestion is also supported by different authors in the field (Monzó 2003; Abril Martí 2006; Sanz-Moreno 2017; Krystallidou et al. 2018), as it implies a conscious involvement in the professional context and a direct relation with the community with whom the students will be working in the future. Nevertheless, from the syllabi of the analysed subjects, it can be deduced that external personnel (professional interpreters, experts on a particular field, etc.) are only used as speakers to give the students some master classes or to present speeches that should be interpreted.

On the other hand, in the trainers' opinion, it is important to have contact with real healthcare equipment and contexts. With that purpose, some of them also use simulation rooms of the Health Faculties at their universities and practise with healthcare students. As a consequence, healthcare interpreting students become familiar with the context and the potential working situation, understand where they have to position themselves, what type of interventions are frequent, etc., and at the same time, they make the healthcare interpreting profession more visible among the future healthcare professionals. The trainers also think that watching real recorded consultations would also be very useful.

Additionally, the trainers explain that they usually include in their teaching difficult situations that a healthcare interpreter may face (culturally embedded dilemmas, emotionally charged situations, etc.) with the aim of preparing the students to face the real problems they will encounter when professionally interpreting.

Finally, according to the syllabi of a few subjects specifically focused on public service interpreting, the possibility to do internships in real contexts (courts, social services departments, hospitals, etc.) is offered. According to the study conducted by Álvaro Aranda and Gutiérrez (2021) previously mentioned, the Spanish universities offering the possibility to do internships related to healthcare interpreting have signed agreements with several healthcare institutions, as for example, outpatient clinics, hospitals, fertility clinics or NGOs which, among other tasks, accompany their users to medical appointments.

5 Conclusions

In the previous pages, the current situation of formal healthcare interpreting training offered at Spanish universities has been generally overviewed. This description may give us some clues about the desirable evolution of this training in the future.

With the professionalisation of healthcare interpreting in mind, several actions should be taken. Among them, raising healthcare professionals' awareness about the importance of working with professional interpreters to improve the quality of healthcare services provided to allophone patients is crucial (Granhagen Jungner et al., 2019; Kletecka-Pulker et al. 2021). Additionally, language access to healthcare should be guaranteed by the law.

This professionalisation process should also be accompanied by training programs at university levels. As explained by Mikkelson (2020: 2), to become "a full-fledged profession in its own right, [healthcare interpreting should be based on] national standards of practice, training programs at accredited colleges and universities, and certification exams as a prerequisite for employment in salaried positions". In this sense, there have been some advances in the last decades in the case of Spain. Currently, and even though healthcare interpreting subjects are not specifically offered in Spanish translation and interpretation degrees, after the Bologna Process, when more flexibility was allowed to the curricula development, Spanish university degrees were to a large extent adapted to the existing needs. Consequently, some changes were made in the curricula to include healthcare interpreting in more broader subjects dealing with public service interpreting and with different names such as social interpreting or intercultural mediation. In this respect, as explained by Vargas Urpí (2016: 97), the diversity in the names of the interpreting subjects may cause some confusion and false expectations for future students. Nevertheless, in our opinion, even though including healthcare interpreting training as part of public service interpreting could be a good way to ensure future professional translators and interpreters have some specific basic competences necessary to carry out this job, this kind of training should be preferably included in specialised postgraduate courses. Bachelor's degrees are intended to be more generalist and postgraduate students are more prepared to delve into particular topics, as they are more mature and usually have previous knowledge and experience.

The problem with the provision of minority languages in the translation and interpretation curricula, which, at the moment, are offered only by very few universities, might be somehow more difficult to tackle. However, a potential solution when there are no qualified trainers to teach interpreting with certain linguistic combinations would be to implement non-language specific courses. Additionally, if healthcare interpreting training is offered through specialised courses which allow the enrolment of students without previous formal recognised university training, people with former ad hoc interpreting experience and speaking minority languages would have the opportunity to obtain a certificate. In any case, this type of curricular design cannot ignore the bidirectionality needed when interpreting in healthcare settings and, consequently, should include some measures as having groups of trainees with the same linguistic combination practising together and supervised, if not by a specialist in the field, at least by lecturers who know the languages involved (Abril Martí 2006: 708).

As for the role of healthcare interpreters, from the data obtained in the focus groups, we may assume that many Spanish trainers and professional interpreters are aware of its specificities and are able to identify the required competences. Moreover, in general, the analysed subjects use adequate methods and contents, but some relevant considerations and improvements could be made.

First of all, healthcare interpreting training should include mixed methodologies, with more time devoted to practical exercises than theoretical classes and a clear closeness to the actual healthcare interpreting practice and its context. In this sense, students should have the possibility to practise with simulations and do internships in real contexts, such as hospitals, clinics, NGOs, etc. Another important methodological aspect consists of the involvement of healthcare professionals in the training, which would not only allow to have contact with the professional community with whom the interpreting trainees will be working in the future, but it would also contribute to the recognition and professionalisation of healthcare interpreting.

As for the contents this training should include, the following should be mentioned:

It may seem obvious, but some of the first and the most important contents are related to the most frequently used interpreting techniques in healthcare settings. These would be onsite and remote liaison interpreting, sight translation and basic techniques for note-taking. Here turn-taking management strategies and pre-interpreting exercises to develop some skills and abilities needed to interpret (such as analysis and synthesis or rephrasing) should also be included.

The interpreting trainees' thematic knowledge should also be developed. Here we refer to the internal procedures and protocols at hospitals, both parties' health system, the most common medical procedures, the typical structure of consultations and medical interviews, the different medical specialities, etc.

As for the languages involved, the different varieties, dialects and registers should be considered. Culture also plays a relevant role and, therefore, cultural patterns related to health, religious beliefs, taboos and traditions should be studied.

Preparing the interpreting trainees to perform documentation and terminology management tasks is essential too.

The knowledge about deontological conduct and the ethical principles should not only be theoretical, but applied, in order to help future healthcare interpreters make reasoned decisions adapted to the context, the participants and the circumstances.

Problem solving skills and interpersonal competences (which prepare the interpreting trainees to negotiate, moderate and explain the interpreter's role) are also indispensable.

Last but not least, healthcare interpreting subjects or courses should include psychological training on how to face difficult situations and prepare the interpreting trainees to give bad news. That is something that has been usually omitted when preparing healthcare interpreters, yet it seems to be gaining importance. Interpreters who operate in healthcare settings work on their own, they do not usually have a team to support them after difficult situations. Therefore, it would be necessary to give them strategies and tools to overcome such situations.

Finally, more materials and resources that are linguistically and culturally adapted to the Spanish context should be developed.

With all these suggestions in mind, the members of the ReACTMe project created a learning platform (available at http://reactme.net/home) containing training resources that could be useful for teaching and learning healthcare interpreting in Spain and organised three short courses (one for trainers and one for trainees) on healthcare interpreting. Additionally, with the aim of raising awareness within the health community, some workshops with healthcare students and professionals about how to work with interpreters were done. Finally, the curriculum of a joint blended module on healthcare interpreting was being developed and will be implemented at the partner universities in the following years.

In conclusion, and according to the literature review and the research conducted within the framework of the ReACTMe project, the need for interpreters who facilitate communication between healthcare professionals and foreign-speaking patients is present, but the recognition of healthcare interpreting as a profession in Spain is far from being reached. In short, we can conclude that healthcare interpreting is currently an under-professionalised activity that, in order to guarantee the allophone patients' rights, should be unambiguously recognised by the Spanish law. Spanish universities have contributed to "the establishment and consolidation of public service interpreting [and healthcare interpreting] as an emergent profession and academic discipline" (Lázaro Gutiérrez and Aranda 2020: 74), but we wonder if it is fair to offer subjects or courses on healthcare interpreting when we cannot guarantee the students' placement in the Spanish labour market. Universities must make an effort to improve their training offer and adapt it to the existing challenges and demands, but only when the institutions and governments provide funding, budgets and support, the implementation of professional healthcare interpreting services will be possible to actually grant the communication rights of the foreign-speaking patients living in or visiting Spain.

References

Abril Martí, María Isabel. 2006. *La Interpretación en los Servicios Públicos: Caracterización como Género, Contextualización y Modelos de Formación. Hacia unas Bases para el Diseño Curricular*. PhD Diss., University of Granada.

Abril Martí, María Isabel, and Anne Martin. 2008. Profesionalizar en la práctica: La competencia en interpretación en los servicios públicos como base para la formación de profesionales. In *Investigación y práctica en traducción e interpretación en los servicios públicos: Desafíos y alianzas*, ed. Valero-Garcés, Carmen, 103–120. Alcalá de Henares: Universidad.

Abril Martí, María Isabel, and Anne Martin. 2011. La barrera de la comunicación como obstáculo en el acceso a la salud de los inmigrantes. In *Actas del I Congreso Internacional sobre Migraciones en Andalucía*, ed. Castaño, García, Francisco Javier, and Nina Kressova, 1521–1534. Granada: Instituto de Migraciones.

Aguayo Arrabal, Natividad. (2019). El encuentro de disciplinas en la formación de traductores: mapa del catálogo oficial de dobles titulaciones en Traducción e Interpretación en España. *Hermeneus, Revista de Traducción e Interpretación* 21: 7–51. https://doi.org/10.24197/her.21.2019.7-51

Álvaro Aranda, Cristina, and Raquel Lázaro Gutiérrez. 2021. La formación en interpretación sanitaria y su camino hacia la profesionalización: un análisis de itinerarios formativos propuestos desde distintas entidades de España. *Panace@* 22(53): 69–71. https://www.tremedica.org/wp-content/uploads/panacea21-53_10_Tribuna_04_AlvaroAranda_LazaroGutierrez.pdf

Angelelli, Claudia V. 2019. Understanding the healthcare setting and its language provision policy. In *Healthcare Interpreting Explained*, 35–36. London/New York: Routledge

Burdeus-Domingo, Noelia, Suzanne Gagnon, Sophie Pointurier, and Yvan Leanza. 2021. Bridges and barriers in public service interpreting training: Instructing non-professional longserving interpreters. *FITISPos International Journal: Public Service Interpreting and Translation* 8: 28–42. https://doi.org/10.37536/FITISPos-IJ.2021.8.1.267

Camacho Sánchez, Fátima. 2019. Formación en traducción e interpretación en los servicios públicos en los programas oficiales de grado impartidos en España *FITISPos International Journal: Public Service Interpreting and Translation*, 6: 235–245

Cross-Cultural Communications. Interpretips. https://www.youtube.com/channel/UCNjL_WcM4BIBw1L0X_ls63Q/featured

Del-Pozo-Triviño, Maribel, (dir.). Linkterpreting. Universidade de Vigo, http://linkterpreting.uvigo.es/

Educaweb. educaweb. Descubre qué estudiar. https://www.educaweb.com/

Foulquié-Rubio, Ana Isabel. 2018. Aproximación a la interpretación en los servicios públicos en la Región de Murcia. In *Panorama de la traducción y la interpretación en los servicios públicos españoles. Una década de cambios, retos y oportunidades*, eds. Foulquié-Rubio, Ana Isabel, Mireia Vargas Urpí, and María Magdalena Fernández Pérez, 137–150. Granada: Comares.

Foulquié-Rubio, Ana Isabel, and Dolores Beteta-Fernández. 2020. Communication issues during triage in a paediatric emergency department. In *Interpreting in legal and healthcare settings: perspectives on research and training*, eds. Ng, Eva N.S. and Ineke H.M. Crezee, 243–262. John Benjamins Publishing Company.

Fundación Universia. Estudios universitarios. https://www.universia.net/es/estudios

Gillies, Andrew. 2004. *Conference interpreting—a new students' companion*. Cracow: Tertium.

Gillies, Andrew. 2013. *Conference interpreting—a students' practice book*. London & New York: Routledge.

Jungner, Granhagen, Elisabet Tiselius Johanna, Klas Blomgren, Kim Lützén, and Pernilla Pergert. 2019. Language barriers and the use of professional interpreters: A national multisite cross-sectional survey in pediatric oncology care. *Acta Oncologica* 58 (7): 1015–1020. https://doi.org/10.1080/0284186X.2019.1594362.

INE. 2019. Spanish national statistics institute. Hostelería y Turismo. https://www.ine.es/dyngs/INEbase/es/categoria.htm?c=Estadistica_P&cid=1254735576863

INE. 2021. Spanish national statistics institute. Demografía y población. https://www.ine.es/index.htm

Interpreting Training Resources. Interpreting training resources. resources for students of conference interpreting. https://interpretertrainingresources.eu/

Kletecka-Pulker, Maria, Sabine Parrag, Klara Doppler, Sabine Völkl-Kernstock, Michael Wagner, and Thomas Wenzel. 2021. Enhancing patient safety through the quality assured use of a low-tech video interpreting system to overcome language barriers in healthcare settings. *Wiener Klinische Wochenschrift* 133: 610–619. https://doi.org/10.1007/s00508-020-01806-7.

Krystallidou, Demi, Myriam Deveugele, Céline Van De Walle, and Evangelia Dougali. 2018. Training doctor-minded interpreters and interpreter-minded doctors: First insights into the benefits of collaborative practice in interpreter training. Interpreting. *An International Journal of Research and Practice in Interpreting* 20 (1): 126–144. https://doi.org/10.1075/intp.00005.kry.

Lázaro Gutiérrez, Raquel, and Cristina Álvaro Aranda. 2020. Public service interpreting and translation in Spain. In *Training public service interpreters and translators: a European perspective*, eds. Štefková, Marketa, Koen Kerremans, and Benjamin Bossaert, 71–87

Martin, Anne. 2015. La formación en interpretación en España: Pasado y presente. *MonTI. Monografías De Traducción E Interpretación* 2: 87–110. https://doi.org/10.6035/MonTI.2015.ne2.3.

Ministerio de Educación, Cultura y Deporte. QUEDU. Qué estudiar y dónde en España. https://www.educacion.gob.es/notasdecorte/busquedaSimple.action

Mikkelson, H. 2020. Development of the medical interpreting profession in the US: A case study. In *Handbook of research on medical interpreting*, ed. Izabel Souza and Effrossyni Fragkou, 1–26. USA: IGI Global.

Monzó, Esther. 2003. Las socializaciones del traductor especializado: El papel de los géneros. *Revista De La Facultad De Lenguas Modernas* 6: 15–29.

Nevado Llopis, Almudena. 2015. The influence of healthcare professionals on medical interpreting recognition and development. *MonTI. Monografías de Traducción e Interpretación*, Special Issue 2. https://doi.org/10.6035/MonTI.2015.ne2.7

Nevado Llopis, Almudena. 2018. Mapa de situación de la traducción y la interpretación en los servicios públicos en Aragón. In *Panorama de la traducción y la interpretación en los servicios públicos españoles. Una década de cambios, retos y oportunidades*, eds. Foulquié Rubio, Ana Isabel, Mireia Vargas Urpí, and María Magdalena Fernández Pérez, 31–46. Granada: Comares.

Nolan, James. 2005. *Interpretation: Techniques and exercises*. Clevedon: Multilingual Matters.

Pérez-Luzardo Díaz, Jessica and María Magdalena Fernández Pérez. 2018. La provisión de la traducción y la interpretación en los servicios públicos de Canarias: retos de un territorio insular. In *Panorama de la traducción y la interpretación en los servicios públicos españoles. Una década de cambios, retos y oportunidades*, eds. Foulquié-Rubio, Ana Isabel, Mireia Vargas Urpí, and María Magdalena Fernández Pérez, 65–81. Granada: Comares.

Plaza Espuña, Isabel, Jordi Grau Bartomeu, Francisco Cegri Lombardo, Cristina Casanovas Guitart, Nuria Domínguez Palicio, Ainhoa Calpe Cristino, Elisabeth Fructuoso González, Montserrat Ochando Aymerich, Jose Ignacio Fernández Martín, Montserrat Rodero Nuño, Manuela Hidalgo Ortiz, Sonia Nar Devi, Aida Chueco Ochando, Mohammad Bashir, and María Petra Pérez-Hervada Maestre. 2015. Barreras idiomáticas en la Atención Primaria de Salud. Percepción de los profesionales sanitarios y bases para estrategias de mejora. In *II Conferencia Internacional de Comunicación en Salud* (23/10/2015). Universidad Carlos III de Madrid. https://e-archivo.uc3m.es/bitstream/handle/10016/21817/barreras_IICICS_2015.pdf?sequence=1&isAllowed=y

ReACTMe. *Research & Action and Training in Medical Interpreting (ReACTMe).* http://reactme.net/home
Registro de Universidades, Centros y Titulaciones, RUCT. TITULACIONES en universidades españolas. Curso 2020–2021. https://www.google.com/url?sa=t&rct=j&q=&esrc=s&source=web&cd=&ved=2ahUKEwi-v8bv69v1AhUTjhQKHVNTDnMQFnoECAIQAQ&url=https%3A%2F%2Fwww.universidades.gob.es%2Fstfls%2Funiversidades%2FEstadisticas%2Fficheros%2Festadisticas_universitarias%2FTitulaciones_uni_espanolas_x_uni-centr-presen_idio-2020.xlsx&usg=AOvVaw0gK6B9dwYWDUK3lz1zkSgm
Román-López, Pablo, María del Mar Palanca-Cruz, Ainhara García-Vergara, Francisco J. Román-López, Sergio Rubio-Carrillo, and Alba Algarte-López. 2015. Barreras comunicativas en la atención sanitaria a la población inmigrante. *Revista Española de Comunicación en Salud* 6(2): 204–212. https://e-revistas.uc3m.es/index.php/RECS/article/view/2939
Sales Salvador, Dora. 2008. Mediación intercultural e interpretación en los servicios públicos. ¿Europa intercultural?. *Pliegos de Yuste. Revista de cultura y pensamiento europeos* 7–8: 77–82. http://www.pliegosdeyuste.eu/n78pliegos/pdf/2008-7-8-77-82.pdf
Sanz Moreno, Raquel. 2017. La inclusión del médico en la formación del intérprete en el ámbito sanitaria. *Revista Digital de Investigación en Docencia Universitaria* 11(2): 203–222. https://doi.org/10.19083/ridu.11.555
Secretaría General Técnica del Ministerio de Universidades. 2021. Datos y cifras del Sistema Universitario Español. Publicación 2020–2021. https://www.universidades.gob.es/stfls/universidades/Estadisticas/ficheros/Datos_y_Cifras_2020-21.pdf
Seleskovitch, Danica, and Marianne Lederer (1989, 2002). *Pédagogie Raisonnée de l'Interprétation.* Brussels & Luxembourg: Didier Érudition.
Tipton, Rebecca, and Olgierda Furmanek. 2016. *Dialogue interpreting: A guide to interpreting in public services and the community.* London/New York: Routledge.
Ugarte Ballester, Xus, and Mireia Vargas Urpí. 2018. La interpretación en los servicios públicos en Catalunya y las Illes Balears. In *Panorama de la traducción y la interpretación en los servicios públicos españoles. Una década de cambios, retos y oportunidades*, eds. Foulquié-Rubio, Ana Isabel, Mireia Vargas Urpí, and María Magdalena Fernández Pérez, 47–64. Granada: Comares.
Valero Garcés, Carmen (2020). Overcoming language barriers in the Spanish healthcare context. In *Interpreting in Legal and Healthcare Settings: Perspectives on research and training*, eds. Ng, Eva N.S. and Ineke H.M. Crezee, 287–312. John Benjamins Publishing Company.
Vargas Urpí, Mireia. 2016."La Difícil Tarea de Dar Respuesta a las Necesidades de Formación en Interpretación en los Servicios Públicos (ISP) en Cataluña: 10 años de Avances y Retrocesos. *FITISPos International Journal: Public Service Interpreting and Translation*, 3: 92–103. http://hdl.handle.net/10230/28259
Zendelel, Rena, Barbara Schouten, Julia Van Weert, and Bas Van Den Putte. 2018. Informal interpreting in general practice: The migrant patient's voice. *Ethnicity and Health* 23 (2): 158–173. https://doi.org/10.1080/13557858.2016.1246939.

Almudena Nevado Llopis holds a PhD in Translation, Society and Communication by Jaume I University. She is a full-time lecturer at the Undergraduate Degrees in Translation and Nursing, and the Master's Degree in Research for Health Sciences at San Jorge University. She is also an associate lecturer at the Master's Degree in Specialized Translation at the University of Vic—Central University of Catalonia. She belongs to the research group Migrations, Interculturality and Human Development (MIDH) and led the Erasmus+ project Research & Action and Training in Medical Interpreting (ReACTMe). She has researched and published in the fields of intercultural communication, public service interpreting, medical interpreting and intercultural mediation.

Ana Isabel Foulquié-Rubio holds a Ph.D. in Translation and Interpreting by the University of Murcia. She is a full-time lecturer of Translation and Interpreting at the University of Murcia where she is in charge of teaching Public Service Interpreting, amongst other courses. She has several publications related to the field of interpreting in public services. She participated in the creation of the Research Group GRETI of the University of Granada, and currently belongs to the Research Group TRADICO of the University of Murcia. She has participated in different research projects such as "Conceptualization and Assessment of Creativity in Translation" (funded by the Seneca Foundation) and "EMOTRA, Translation and Emotions" (funded by the Spanish Ministry of Education). She participated in the ReACTMe Project (funded by the European Commission).

Interpreter-Mediated End-of-Life Encounters in Spain: Mapping the Spanish Situation Based on Healthcare Providers' Input

Elena Pérez Estevan

1 Introduction

Public Service Interpreting (PSI) or Community Interpreting takes place as a social need in today's multilingual society to enable people to communicate within the public institutions including educational, legal or medical settings. Although public service interpreters have existed throughout human history, they have received more attention by academia since the twentieth century, as Iliescu Gheorghiu (2022) points out in the ENTI encyclopaedia[1]:

> Community or public service interpreting is a relatively recent coinage (end of 20th century) referring to an interlinguistic and intercultural communication that serves the community and takes place in and for the public services, be it legal (police, asylum, prisons), medical or educational.

Topics such as quality, ethics, working conditions, user expectations or interpreters' role in PSI have been approached by research.

Quality has been a complex concept to define in interpreting in general and in PSI. Barik (1971) and Gerver (2002) started to research errors as a quality criterion in interpreting; Gile (1985), Bühler (1986) and Garzone (2003) introduced users' expectations in quality research and Pöchhacker (2001) added healthcare professionals' expectations, to name just a few. In the last decade, other criteria have been addressed in terms of quality like training (Camacho Sánchez 2019), the level of professionalization (Enriquez Raído et al. 2020) or users' comprehension (Amato 2018) and trust (Aguilar Solano 2020), among others. Notwithstanding the fact that

[1] An open encyclopaedia of the Iberian Association for Translation and Interpreting Studies (AIETI) https://www.aieti.eu/enciclopedia/presentacion/.

E. Pérez Estevan (✉)
University of Alicante, Alicante, Spain
e-mail: elena.perezestevan@ua.es

R. Lázaro Gutiérrez and C. Álvaro Aranda (eds.), *New Trends in Healthcare Interpreting Studies*, New Frontiers in Translation Studies,
https://doi.org/10.1007/978-981-99-2961-0_8

quality has been the focus of many researchers, a consensus on what "good quality" means has not been reached yet as stated by Pöchhacker (2015: 333):

> Interpreting scholars do not have a single, universal and agreed definition of quality that could be applied to all interpreting events across historical, cultural and social contexts. Multiple, and sometimes even contradictory, definitions highlight different aspects of quality, depending on the object of the study.

Research on the public service interpreter's role has had a broad impact in the literature and continues to be related to the discussion on interpreters' visibility in different settings. Some authors argued that the interpreter should remain neutral to convey the message faithfully for both parties (Garber 2000; Mesa 2000) and, in the opposite view, the interpreter can be seen as playing an active role as a communication 'co-constructor' (Wadensjö 2001), patient 'advocacy' (Roberts 1997) or 'cultural mediator' (Jalbert 1998). In between these opposing views, some authors described different roles for the interpreter as for example the 'family support role' of the interpreter for the families in his research on paediatric units (Leanza 2005) or the 'patient navigators' role' of the interpreter for patients with difficulties accessing healthcare services (Crezee 2013). Regarding the complexity describing the role of the public service interpreter, Bancroft (2015) mentioned confidentiality, accuracy and impartiality as essential standards for interpreters independent of the role adopted. In the last decade, role has also been analysed based on the backdrop against which the interpreter is working such as domestic violence (Pozo Triviño 2017), prisons (Baixauli Olmos 2013), and asylum procedures (Bergunde et al. 2017).

The (professional) status of interpreter has also been studied in terms of role and quality. Flores et al. (2012) compared the performance of professional interpreters, ad-hoc interpreters and non-interpreter-mediated situations in 57 encounters in visits to the emergency department in Massachusetts, concluding that the percentage of errors with potential consequences was significantly lower in the case of professional interpreters. The authors also concluded that trained interpreters were less likely to make mistakes or at least less serious ones in terms of consequences for quality and patient safety.

Foulquié Rubio (2018) described the situation in a Spanish region where healthcare providers have difficulties communicating the diagnosis and treatment to non-Spanish speaking patients when they use ad hoc interpreters.

The use of children as interpreters in healthcare (Child Language Brokers, CLB) has been addressed from the point of view of the negative consequences for both parties (Hall and Sam 2008; Antonini 2010) and the effects on educational and psychological development of these CLBs (Orellana et al. 2003; Weisskirch 2007; Orellana 2009; Cline et al. 2017).

Regarding PSI in Spain, the legislation is far from the desired professionalization level existing in other countries such as United Kingdom, United States, Australia or Sweden. In the volume edited by Foulquié Rubio, Vargas-Urpi and Fernández Pérez (2018) mapping the situation of PSI Spain, it is stated that the legislation does not guarantee the access to medical services to non-Spanish speaking patients because, even though they have the right to be appropriately informed, interpreting services are not provided by law (*ibid.*, 3). Hence, "public service interpreting in Spain remains an under-professionalised activity" (Lázaro Gutiérrez and Álvaro Aranda 2021: 71).

Within the healthcare interpreting context, the present paper aims to go beyond and map the situation of interpreter-mediated end-of-life and grief encounters in Spain. Hence, healthcare expectations of the interpreters' role in end-of-life encounters is analysed and interpreters' emotional support is approached. This research emphasizes the need to use debriefing sessions to let interpreters vent their emotions and share difficult experiences after being exposed to traumatic situations which may affect their emotion management. Nonetheless, despite the importance of this topic in PSI, not many studies have analysed this specific field from the healthcare providers' perspective on which this study focuses.

Section 3 introduces the methods used in this research, and, in Sect. 4, results of the survey and interviews are discussed. Finally, Sect. 5 will be devoted to conclusions.

2 Brief Reflection on the Impact of Communication Barriers in End-Of-Life and Grief Encounters

End-of-life contexts in this study cover palliative care visits and grief therapies, either individual or group, after the loss of a loved one. Hofmeister et al. (2018: 17) described the aim of palliative care as "to improve quality of life of patients and families through the prevention and relief of suffering". Grief is a natural response to loss and it commonly involves emotional suffering, unexpected emotions and sadness. Coping with the loss of a loved one can become a stressful experience. Hence grief therapies and/or grief support groups can help the bereaved process the loss. Costa (2020) differentiates multilingual therapies from monolingual due to the influence of languages in how the bereaved feels the emotions, expresses them and experiences the world because "the language we speak influences not only the way we see the word around us, but also the way we see and think about ourselves" (Marian and Kaushanskaya 2004: 198 *cfr.* Costa 2020: 2).

Despite communication being essential in end-of-life contexts, interpreter-mediated encounters in palliative care visits at home and interpreter-mediated grief encounters have received scant attention in Spain. Consequently, language barriers lead to miscommunication and pose challenges on the delivery of palliative care and grief support.

Some studies highlight the situation of foreign patients who experience unequal access to healthcare services (Hilfinger et al. 2009; Annete and Sakellariou 2017), misdiagnoses (Karliner et al. 2010) or medication complications (Bowen 2015). Miscommunication can also affect pain control and cause more physical and emotional suffering. It also leads to confusion and lack of planning (Nelson 2018).

Although death and loss are universal experiences, attitudes, circumstances and understandings of grief are different from one human to another (Neymeyer and Smigelsky 2018). Recently, the pandemic situation due to COVID-19 has also affected how people see, think and experience death and loss (Alonso Fernández 2021; Valero Garcés 2021; Pérez Estevan 2022).

Communication barriers are perceived by some healthcare providers as a source of stress (Bernard et al. 2006; Fiabane et al. 2012) and they have negative implications for both parties, patients and healthcare professionals, satisfaction, safety and quality of healthcare services (Johnstone and Kanitsaki 2006; Aboumatar et al. 2015; Al Shamsi et al. 2020).

Silva et al. (2016) analysed the influence of professional interpreters on the delivery of palliative services. They conducted a systematic review of the literature from 1960 to 2014. Their findings show that when interpreters were not available, patients had worse quality care discussions.

Stress has also been associated, among other reasons, to losing power control as pointed out by Siyu Wu and Rawal (2017: 6) "if you don't have a voice, you are powerless", as well as by Costa (2020: 5):

> An additional theme connected with power is the counsellor or psychotherapist's anxiety about not understanding what is being said in the therapy room, where understanding and communication are the cornerstones of the work.

Stress has also been analysed in the interpreter's performance and emotional management. The continuous involvement of the interpreter in sensitive situations such as palliative care delivery and being the voice of emotionally affected people can lead to interpreters' emotional distress and difficulties in decision making (Hsieh and Nicodemus 2015).

Within the context of emotions, empathy plays an important role. Edlins and Dolamore (2018) defined empathy as the ability to recognize, understand and respond to others' feelings. Although empathy is considered a central factor for a successful doctor-patient interaction, its limits remain unclear, as well as the question whether empathy is innate, learned or a combination of both. Valero Garcés and Alcalde Peñalver (2021) carried out a systematic review of the studies related to empathy in public service interpreting from 2000 to 2020. They distinguished between studies that focus on empathy and studies that do not focus on it but contain references to it. Their findings reveal that empathy has been approached from different perspectives (interpreter' role, code of conduct and different settings) but there are discrepancies between the standards and codes of ethics and how empathy is managed in practice.

Empathy has been related to vicarious trauma and compassion fatigue in PSI. Vicarious trauma is experienced after having been constantly exposed to traumatic experiences of others. Although the interpreter has not experienced the traumatic event first hand, he/she feels an intense shift in worldview (Vigor 2012; Darroch and Dempsey 2016). Compassion fatigue means a profound emotional exhaustion which negatively affects the ability to be empathetic with the patient (Beauvais et al. 2017). Vicarious trauma and compassion fatigue have been identified as predictors of burnout for interpreters who work with asylum seekers, refugees and torture survivors (Teegen and Goennenwein 2002; Shlesinger, 2005; Splevins et al. 2010; Kindermann et al. 2017).

From the perspective of improving public service interpreters' wellbeing few studies have been carried out. A pilot study on the provision of remote self-care support for interpreters working in sensitive contexts was performed by Costa et al. (2020). Their conclusions indicated an increase in self-care and confidence and a successful way of processing difficult experiences in terms of emotions. Another experimental training course about emotional management was designed for eleven public service interpreters who suffered from anxiety or depression because of their job (Bruno and Iborra Cuéllar 2021). They concluded that the intervention, consisting of 10 sessions, was successful in terms of increasing emotional intelligence. Costa (2017) goes beyond and proposes a method of supervision for interpreters either one-to-one or in a group (2020) with three functions: The first is "reparative", to allow interpreters to improve their performance; the second is "reflexive", to vent their feelings and listen to other interpreters' experiences, and the third is the "responsive" function to help interpreters find solutions to problems that arise from the institutions' organization or systems (*vid.* Costa 2020: 90–95). This approach responds to her concern about interpreters' emotional management:

> Therapists need to think about how we can help interpreters to manage the emotional challenges of the work; managers should ensure there is funding to provide this help included in the overall cost of interpreting services. It is an additional cost in the short term, but in the long term there is cost saving because there will be fewer absences and resulting cancelled appointments (Costa 2020: 60).

In a country such as Spain where the interpreting profession is not subject to specific regulations, finding the balance between being empathetic and being able to manage emotions properly is a difficult task for the interpreter working in end-of-life contexts.

3 Methods

The present paper investigates Spanish healthcare providers' perceptions and expectations of the interpreters' needs and tasks in palliative care units and in grief therapies. To approach this unaddressed area, we use a quantitative method (a survey) and a qualitative tool (in-depth interviews) to complement the results obtained in the quantitative analysis.

The data discussed in the following sections is part of a doctoral research project focused on interpreting performance in end-of-life contexts from the perspective of all parties involved. However, this paper will focus on healthcare providers' views.

The first objective addressed here is examining the importance given to communication in end-of-life context from the perspective of healthcare providers. It also considers healthcare providers' perspectives and expectations of the interpreters' tasks in interpreter-mediated end-of-life situations.

Secondly, we analyse if briefing and debriefing sessions could be a useful tool to approach interpreters' emotional wellbeing in end-of-life contexts within the Spanish context of interpreting not being fully recognized legally speaking. Within the emotions' research, respondents are also questioned if knowing each other (healthcare provider and interpreter) from previous collaborations would have an impact on the debriefing session.

To fulfil these objectives and to map the interpreter-mediated end-of-life situation in Spain, data was collected via a survey that was distributed electronically. The survey consisted of 29 questions. In some of them, participants could provide short answers, whereas other questions asked respondents to fill out a Likert scale containing 10 gradings of importance.

The informants of the survey are healthcare providers who work in hospitals or medical centres, but not necessarily in palliative care units or grief therapies. However, they all have been immersed in end-of-life situations in their departments (cardiology, intensive care unit, nursing, primary care, oncology and organ donation department). To map the situation of interpreting in end-of-life contexts, the second part of the analysis focuses on interviewing professionals involved in the delivery of palliative care at home and professionals who conduct grief therapies either individual or in support groups. For this aim, we carried out 71 in-depth interviews. Consent forms were obtained and registered appropriately.

4 Results and Discussion

4.1 Results of the Survey About Healthcare Providers' Perceptions and Expectations

The total sample of informants consists of 205 healthcare providers. 60% of them have worked with interpreters, whereas 40% have not. Of the 60% who have worked with interpreters, 40% of the respondents had experience with ad-hoc interpreters and the other 20% with professional interpreters.

The central focus of the first series of questions for healthcare providers was to know their opinion about the importance of communication with patients at the end of their live and with their relatives and with bereaved people. They were given a ten-point Likert scale from 0 to 10 (being 0 unimportant and 10 extremely important). 175 out of 205 participants responded with 10 points to the question of communicating with the patient; 143 gave 10 points to the question about relatives and 184 marked the maximum level of importance when communicating with the bereaved.

If we convert these numbers in percentages, communication with patients at the end of life was considered extremely important by 85% of participants. The same level of importance was given to communication with relatives by 75% of respondents. Finally, communication with the bereaved was indicated with 10 points by 90% of participants. The rest of answers varied from important, moderately important and very important, that is to say, from 6 to 9 points in the scale.

Participants were also questioned about their expectations of interpreters working in end-of-life contexts. Seven criteria were given:

Table 1 shows a very high level of agreement from respondents regarding the importance given to the criteria related to what healthcare providers expect from interpreters. In fact, maximum percentages from participants are for the option 'extremely important' followed by 'very important'. Confidentiality has the highest percentage for the option 'extremely important' followed by trust and respect of others' feelings and emotions. These responses show healthcare providers give more importance to tasks in line with emotions rather than linguistic areas. A reason is deduced from the results: healthcare providers do not consider themselves experts to judge linguistic criteria so that they give more importance to parameters related to doctor-patient relationship.

The second series of questions was addressed at examining the importance given to briefing and debriefing sessions between healthcare providers and interpreters. Results are presented in the following Table 2.

The responses presented in Table 2 underscore the importance given by participants to briefing and debriefing sessions with interpreters. Healthcare providers pointed to the view that briefing is needed to get a better understanding of the participants' role, to prepare for the encounter in terms of how to deliver the information, especially bad news, discuss care plan or treatment, if possible, and/or the referral to palliative care if needed, and create an atmosphere of trust which sometimes becomes essential to reassure and help patients suffering from emotional distress.

According to the second objective (i.e., whether briefing and debriefing sessions could be a useful tool for interpreters' emotional wellbeing in end-of-life contexts), responses to why debriefing was important indicated opening a space to discuss

Table 1 Respondents' expectations of interpreters' tasks (in percentages)

	Slightly	Moderate	Very	Extremely
Completeness of information	6	10	20	64
Correctly translated information	4.5	10	20.5	65
Familiarity with terminology	10	20	25	45
Fluency	13	20	22.5	44.5
Respect of others' feelings and emotions	2	10	18	70
Trust	2	12	16	70
Confidentiality	0	6.5	6.5	87

Table 2 Respondents' perspectives of the importance of briefing and debriefing sessions with interpreters (in percentages)

	Moderate	Very	Extremely
Briefing	0	45	55
Debriefing	15	65	20

the outcome of the consultation and to express participants' feelings and emotions, especially after a patient's death.

All healthcare providers agreed that debriefing sessions would be ideal for the interpreter to vent emotions and feelings because briefing sessions are normally dedicated to prepare for the visit.

Following our aims, we also examined if there is an impact on the seven criteria if the healthcare provider and the interpreter have worked together in previous collaborations. Informants were asked to provide their opinion by considering if it may have a positive or negative effect or if it has no effect at all. Responses are presented in Table 3.

Table 3 shows a high consensus on the positive impact of knowing each other in terms of the criteria given. Trust and less stressful situations have received the highest positive impact percentage (95%) followed by respect of others' feelings and emotions and empathy and correctly translated information (85%). Even though the criteria 'a better understanding of the patient's social context' and 'a better understanding of the patient's emotions and feelings' have obtained high results to positive impact, they have obtained the highest answer to negative impact choice among the others (13% and 15% percentages, respectively). The explanation they gave for negative impact option was related to difficulties establishing role boundaries in interpreter-mediated sessions. The results indicate in the opinion of informants, linguistic criteria such as accuracy and correctly translated information have the highest percentage of no effect (18% for the first one and 10% for the second one). These figures may indicate that they do not consider they have sufficient ability to evaluate these two items as deducted from the previous question.

Finally, the last question of the survey (i.e., mapping the Spanish situation of interpreter-mediated end-of-life sessions) was if the respondents know where to find a professional interpreter. 67% of the informants answered they did not, whereas the other 33% indicated they did.

Table 3 Respondents' perspectives of the impact of previous collaborations (in percentages)

	Positive	Negative	No effect
Accuracy	80	2	18
Correctly translated information	85	2	10
Respect of others' feelings and emotions and empathy	85	10	5
Better understanding of the patient's social context	84	13	3
Better understanding of the patient's emotions and feelings	80	15	5
Trust	95	5	0
Less stressful situations	95	5	0

4.2 Results of In-Depth Interviews with Healthcare Providers About Their Perceptions and Expectations

This qualitative study was carried out in 2021 containing 71 in-depth interviews, with healthcare providers who have trained as psychotherapists as well and who work in home palliative care units[2] and in grief support associations, to complement the results obtained in the survey. The aim of this study was to provide insight into healthcare providers' perceptions of interpreting at the end of life in the patient's home in Spain to overview this daily practice outside a hospital setting as some patients often decide to receive palliative care at home.

The initial assumption was: if professional interpreting in hospital settings in Spain often lacks regulation and awareness by some healthcare providers, the number of professional interpreters in non-hospital settings, palliative care at home and grief associations, will decrease.

The first group of informants included 15 healthcare providers who work in palliative care units in hospital and at patients' homes. The second group was made up of 9 informants who work in grief therapies or support groups for the bereaved in different Spanish associations. The third group includes three healthcare providers who work in grief therapies and support groups and in palliative care. Finally, the fourth group is made up of 44 healthcare providers who work in palliative services at home.

Only 5 out of 71 interviewees had worked with professional interpreters when delivering palliative care at the patient's home because the patient had hired the interpreter. These 5 informants belonged to the first group (healthcare providers in hospital). Taking time to know the patient and the family and their emotions and feelings, having important discussions about the state of the patient, planning the final stage period, knowing the patient's desires and preferences for information and decision making were positive consequences noticed by healthcare professionals.

The remaining 10 informants of the first group, plus the 44 of the fourth group (54 in total) had worked with ad-hoc interpreters such as relatives, friends or neighbours of the limited Spanish proficiency patient. Among them, 39 interviewees discussed their perceptions when working with ad-hoc interpreters and 15 healthcare providers experienced the use of children as interpreters for their relatives who were at end of life.

The following Fig. 1 contains the data on healthcare providers' experiences working with interpreters:

Healthcare providers' perceptions of ad-hoc interpreters included difficulties discussing patient state, emotions and feelings. They also experienced communication breakdowns and divergences between non-verbal communication of the patient and verbal communication of ad-hoc interpreters.

Despite these negative perceptions, one interviewee had a positive experience working with an ad-hoc interpreter who was a Chinese friend of the patient. This

[2] In Spain, these units are called *Unidad de Cuidados Paliativos a Domicilio, Unidad de Cuidados Paliativos Domiciliario* and *Unidad de Hospitalización a domicilio.*

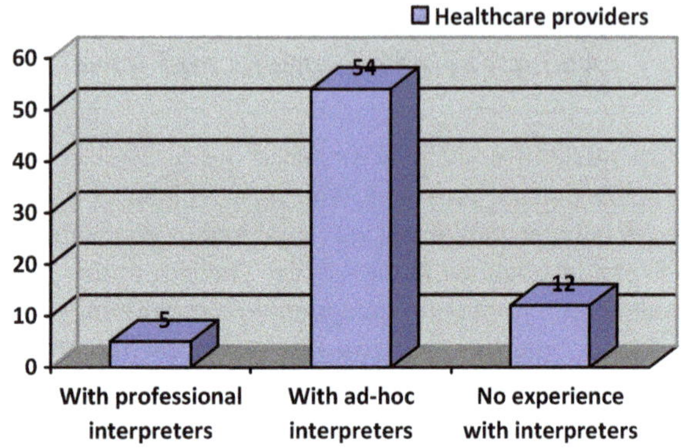

Fig. 1 Healthcare providers' experience working with interpreters

person had helped the patient and healthcare professionals in hospital in previous sessions and she interpreted as well at home. The informant reported a good command of Spanish from the ad-hoc interpreter. In addition, sharing the patient's culture was a positive aspect highlighted because it helped them to understand the patient's view of death and rituals.

As a consequence of the use of child language brokers, these 15 professionals stated the impossibility of talking about emotions, dealing with important matters for them such as pain management, side effects of medication and the inability to mention anything about the death circumstances or grief-related topics. They also mentioned the stress and the burden caused to the child language brokers because they take responsibilities in situations out of their control which may entail complications for their grieving processes. These healthcare professionals and the ones who worked with ad-hoc interpreters often found cases of conspiracy of silence[3] which led to healthcare dehumanization and communication failure.

Yet, an informant shared a satisfactory experience when working with a patient who was seriously ill at the final stage and her 22-year-old daughter helped them with communication. From this interviewee's perception, a good relationship between the patient and her daughter benefited the emotional openness.

None of the participants in the second or the third group had worked with interpreters, which means that professionals working in grief therapies or support groups have not been contacted by limited Spanish-proficiency patients. During their interviews, 10 participants out of 12 (the total sample of the second and third group) stated that they consider non-Spanish speaking bereaved people do not know about their services. Hence, hiring an interpreter was not discussed, although 2 of them mentioned that on one occasion they were contacted by an ad hoc interpreter (a friend and a relative) to find out about their services. In the end, bereaved people did not receive grief therapy due to language barriers. Neither of these 2 providers were aware of where to find a professional interpreter. As a matter of fact, all interviewees were questioned whether they knew where to find a professional interpreter and none

[3] Conspiracy of silence in palliative care "generally involves family members and healthcare teams who withhold full or partial information from the patient" (Lemus Riscanevo et al. 2019: 27).

of them did. Six of them thought they could ask the social worker of their medical centres or hospitals.

Participants were also questioned about their expectations of professional interpreters' tasks working in end-of-life contexts according to the seven criteria suggested in the survey presented in the previous section. All participants expected completeness of information and its correct translation, familiarity with terminology and fluency. Informants also rated as extremely important the respect of others' feelings and emotions, trust and confidentiality. They also added that if the interpreter was familiar with how a palliative unit works and had a close communication with the patient and family and the palliative team it would be a bonus. Some of them stated that they would prefer to always use the same interpreter for a patient if possible because they experienced situations in which the interpreter, even though it was an ad-hoc one, has been a different one on some occasions and the outcome was chaotic in terms of organization, care and communication.

Within the context of communicating emotions, if briefing and debriefing sessions would be useful to let interpreters vent emotions and feelings was also discussed in the interviews. For informants of the second and third group, a briefing session before the grief therapy would be essential due to the sensitive topics and the exposure to traumatic experiences that they are not aware of the impact on the interpreter. In the debriefing sessions they would focus on interpreter's wellbeing, emotions and feelings. The rest of informants consider debriefing sessions more useful and possibly successful to vent emotions and feelings because the briefing sessions are normally used to discuss patient care and plan.

These findings strengthen the idea that despite the importance of communication in end-of-life contexts, the reality shows that professional interpreters are not often used to interpret at patient's home because healthcare professionals are not aware of where to find professional interpreters unless the patient hires them. From the healthcare providers' perspective, the patients' economic situation is involved when choosing a professional or an ad-hoc interpreter.

5 Conclusions

The aim of this study was to map the Spanish situation of interpreter-mediated end-of-life situations based on healthcare providers' experiences. The survey and in-depth interviews allowed us to have an overview of the current situation on the topic of the interpreters' role and tasks in end-of-life encounters from healthcare providers. It also enabled us to reach the second objective: an approach to the interpreter's wellbeing by exploring if briefing and debriefing could be used to vent emotions.

The results of both studies support the need of professional interpreters in the end-of-life context: in palliative units in hospital settings and at patients' home as well as in grief therapies –individual and support groups, to enhance communication with limited Spanish proficiency patients, relatives and healthcare providers.

Expectations of interpreters from the perspective of healthcare providers, in order of rated importance, include confidentiality, trust, respect of others' feelings and emotions, correctly translated information, completeness of information, familiarity with terminology and fluency. In the interviews, informants added familiarity with the functioning of a palliative unit and availability of the interpreter as important factors for them.

This study has corroborated the need for briefing and debriefing sessions. Participants considered briefing as important for fostering greater understanding of the interpreter's role, preparing the encounter, discussing the care plan and treatment and enhancing trust among the team. Informants also underline the importance and usability of debriefing sessions to serve as support for interpreters to vent their feelings, process difficult experiences, hear others' experiences and perspectives and cope with emotion management. As observed, healthcare providers consider that getting to know the interpreter improves trust, accuracy, respect of others' feelings and emotions and empathy. Moreover, it helps a better understanding of the patient's social context and emotional state, and it leads to less stressful situations.

The sample of participants was 276 in total (205 respondents to the survey and 71 in-depth interviews) and just 25% of them would know where to find a professional interpreter despite the need for them in the area of study. The current research shows the situation in practice where healthcare providers face communicative barriers due to the absence of professional interpreters unless the patient hires them. The economic situation of the patient influences the choice to hire a professional interpreter from healthcare providers' impressions and experience.

Most limited Spanish proficiency patients are helped by ad-hoc interpreters specially when palliative care is delivered at the patient's home. The use of child language brokers is categorized as a negative practice from the perspective of participants because it poses difficulties in discussing the patient's emotional state and leads to communication breakdowns and divergences. This situation emphasizes the need for specific legislation to professionalize public service interpreting and to reach standards of role, quality and ethics in different contexts such as end-of-life interpreting.

Being aware of the limitations of this study, it can be seen as a starting point to continued contribution to research on interpreting in end-of-life encounters and grief therapies. Further research on vicarious trauma, compassion fatigue and burnout is needed to raise awareness of the importance of good mental health and wellbeing for interpreters involved in end-of-life contexts.

References

Aboumatar, Hanan, Bickey Chang, Jad Al Danaf, Mohammad Shaear, Ruth Namuyinga, Sathyanarayanan Elumalai, Jill Marsteller and Peter Pronovost. 2015. Promising practices for achieving patient-centred hospital care: A national study of high-performing US hospitals. *Medical Care* 53(9): 758–767.

Aguilar Solano, María. 2020. Triangulation and trustworthiness. Advancing research on public service interpreting through qualitative case study methodologies. *Fitispos International Journal* 7: 31–52.

Al Shamsi, Hilal, Abdullah Almutairi, Sulaiman Al Mashrafi and Talib Al Kalbani. 2020. Implications of language barriers for healthcare: a systematic review. *Oman Medical Journal* 35(2): 1–7.

Alonso Fernández, Marcos. 2021. Beyond health and wealth: the impact of COVID-19 and anti-COVID-19 measures on the narrative dimension of human life. *Academia Letters*, Article 660.

Amato, Amalia. 2018. Challenges and solutions. Some paradigmatic examples. In *Handbook of remote interpreting—SHIFT in Orality*, ed. Amato, Amalia, Nicoletta Spinolo and María Jesús González Rodríguez, 79–101. University of Bologna.

Annete, Floyd, and Dikaios Sakellariou. 2017. Healthcare access for refugee women with limited literacy: Layers of disadvantage. *International Journal for Equity in Health* 16 (1): 195.

Antonini, Rachele. 2010. The study of child language brokering: Past, current and emerging research. *MediAzioni* 10. http://mediazioni.sitlec.unibo.it. ISSN 1974-4382.

Baixauli Olmos, Lluís. 2013. A description of interpreting in prisons. Mapping the setting through an ethical lens. In *Interpreting in a changing landscape*, ed. Schäffner, Christina, Krzysztof Kredens and Yvonne Fowler, 45–60. Selected papers from Critical Link 6. Amsterdam: John Benjamins.

Bancroft, Marjory. 2015. Community interpreting: a profession rooted in social justice. In *The routledge handbook of interpreting*, ed. Mikkelson, Holly and Renée Jourdenais, 217-235. London: Routledge.

Barik, Henry. 1971. A description of various types of omissions, additions and errors of translation encountered in simultaneous interpretation. *Meta* 16 (4): 199–210.

Beauvais, Audrey, Michael Andreychik, and Linda A. Henkel. 2017. The role of emotional intelligence and empathy in compassionate nursing care. *Mindfulness & Compassion* 2: 92–100.

Bergunde, Annika, Sonja Pöllabauer, and Iris Topolovec, eds. 2017. *Handbook for interpreters in Asylum procedures*. Wien: ONU.

Bernard, Andrew, Misty Whitaker, Myrna Ray, Anna Rockich, Marietta Barton-Baxter, Stephen Barnes, Bernard Boulanger, Betty Tsuei and Paul Kearney. 2006. Impact of language barrier on acute care medical professionals is dependent upon role. *Journal of Professional Nursing* 22(6): 355–358.

Bowen, Sarah. 2015. The impact of language barriers on patient safety and quality of care. *Société Santé en français*, 1–53.

Bruno, Luana and Alejandro Iborra Cuéllar. 2021. Un programa de intervención para fomentar la gestión emocional en un grupo de intérpretes sociales. *Fitispos International Journal* 8(1): 43–65. https://doi.org/10.37536/FITISPos-IJ.2021.8.1.269.

Bühler, Hildegund. 1986. Linguistic (semantic) and extra-linguistic (pragmatic) criteria for the evaluation of conference interpretation and interpreters. *Multilingua* 5 (4): 231–235.

Camacho Sánchez, Fátima. 2019. Training in public service translation and interpreting in BA degree programmes taught in Spain. *Fitispos International Journal* 6: 235–245.

Cline, Tony, Sarah Crafter, Guida Abreu and Lindsay O'Dell. 2017. Child language brokers' representations of parent-child relationships. In *Non-professional Interpreting and Translating: State of the art and future of an emerging field of research*, ed. Rachelle Antonini, Letizia Cirillo, Linda Rossato and Ira Torresi, 281–294. Benjamins Translation Library.

Costa, Beverley. 2020. *Other tongues: Psychological therapies in a multilingual world*. Monmouth: PCCS Books.

Costa, Beverley, Raquel Lázaro Gutiérrez and Tom Rausch. 2020. Self-care as an ethical responsibility: a pilot study on support provision for interpreter in human crises. *Translation and Interpreting Studies* 15(1): 36–56.
Costa, Beverley. 2017. The strength and the stress of triangles: Support and supervision for interpreters and therapists. In *Psychological therapy with torture survivors in Exile; A human rights approach*, ed. Boyles, Jake, 331–350. Monmouth: PCCS Books.
Crezee, Ineke. 2013. *Introduction to healthcare for interpreters and translators*. Amsterdam: John Benjamins Publishing Company.
Darroch, Emma, and Raymond Dempsey. 2016. Interpreters' experiences of transferential dynamics, vicarious traumatisation, and their need for support and supervision: A systematic literature review. *The European Journal of Counselling Psychology*. https://doi.org/10.5964/EJCOP.V41 2.76.
Edlins, Mariglynn, and Stephanie Dolamore. 2018. Ready to serve the public? The role of empathy in public service education programs. *Journal of Public Affairs Education* 24 (7): 1–21.
Fiabane, Elena, Ines Giorgi, Daniele Musian, Cinzia Sguazzin and Piergiorgio Argentero. 2012. Occupational stress and job satisfaction of healthcare staff in rehabilitation units. La medicina del lavoro 103(6): 482–492.
Enríquez Raído, Vanessa, Ineke Crezee and Quintin Ridgeway. 2020. Professional, ethical and policy dimensions of public service interpreting and translation in New Zeland. *TIS (Translation and Interpreting Studies)* 15(1): 15–35.
Foulquié Rubio, Ana Isabel. 2018. Aproximación a la interpretación en los servicios públicos en la región de Murcia [An approach to public service interpreting in the Region of Murcia]. In Panorama de la traducción y la interpretación en los servicios públicos españoles. Una década de cambios, retos y oportunidades, ed. Foulquié Rubio, Ana Isabel, Mireia Vargas Urpi and Magdalena Fernández Pérez, 137–150. Granada: Comares.
Flores, Glenn, Milagros Abreu, Cara Pizzo Barone, Richard Bachur and Hua Lin. 2012. Errors of medical interpretation and their potential clinical consequences: A comparison of professional versus ad hoc versus no interpreters. *Annals of Emergency* 60(5): 545–553.
Garber, Nathan. 2000. Community interpretation: a personal view. In: *The critical link 2: interpreters in the community*, ed. Roberts, Roda, Silvana E. Carr, Diana Abraham and Aideen Dofour, 9–20. Amsterdam/Filadelfia: John Benjamins.
Garzone, Giuliana Elena. 2003. Reliability of quality criteria evaluation in survey research. In *La evaluación de la calidad en interpretación: Investigación*, ed. Collados Aís, Ángela, Mª Manuela Fernández Sánchez and Daniel Gile, 23–30. Granada: Comares.
Gerver, David. 2002. The effects of source language presentation rate on the performance of simultaneous conference interpreters. In *The interpreting studies reader*, ed. Franz Pöchhacker and Miriam Shlesinger, 53–66. London/New York: Routledge.
Gile, Daniel. 1985. La sensibilité aux écarts de langue et la sélection d'informateurs dans l'analyse d'erreurs: Une expérience. *The Incorporated Linguist* 24 (1): 29–32.
Hall, Nigel, and Sylvia Sam. 2008. Language brokering as young people's work: Evidence from Chinese adolescents in England. *Language and Education* 21 (1): 16–30.
Hilfinger Messias, Deanne Karen, Liz McDowell, Robin Dawson. 2009. Language interpreting as social justice work: perspectives of formal and informal healthcare interpreters. *ANS Advances in Nursing Science* 32(2): 128–143.
Hofmeister, Mark, Ally Memedovich, Laura Dowsett, Laura Sevick, Tamara McCarron, Eldon Spackman, Tania Stafinski, Devidas Menon, Tom Noseworthy and Fiona Clement. 2018. Palliative care in the home: a scoping review of study quality, primary outcomes, and thematic component analysis. *BMC Palliative Care* 41: 17–41.
Hsieh, Elaine, and Brenda Nicodemus. 2015. Conceptualizing emotion in healthcare interpreting: A normative approach to interpreters' emotion work. *Patient Education and Counselling* 98: 1474–1481.

Iliescu Gheorghiu, Catalina. 2022. Community interpreting. In Enciclopedia de Traducción e Interpretación (ENTI) de la Asociación Ibérica de Estudios de Traducción e Interpretación (AIETI), ed. Muñoz, Ricardo and Javier Franco. https://www.aieti.eu/enciclopedia/.

Jalbert, Martin. (1998). Travailler avec un interprète en consultation psychiatrique. P.R.I.S.M.E. 8(3): 94–111.

Johnstone, Megan Jane, and Olga Kanitsaki. 2006. Culture, language, and patient safety: Making the link. *International Journal for Quality in Healthcare* 18 (5): 383–388.

Karliner, Leah, Sue E. Kim, David Meltzer and Andrew Auerbach. 2010. Influence of language barriers on outcomes of hospital care for general medicine inpatients. *Journal of Hospital Medicine* 5(5): 276–282.

Kindermann, David, Carolin Schmid, Cassandra Derreza-Greeven, Daniel Huhn, Rupert Maria Kohl, Florian Junne, Maritta Schleyer, Judith Daniels, Beate Ditzen, Wolfgang Herzog and Christoph Nikendei. 2017. Prevalence of and risk factors for secondary traumatization in interpreters for refugees: a cross-sectional study. Psychopathology 50(4): 262–272. https://doi.org/10.1159/000477670.

Lázaro Gutiérrez, Raquel and Cristina Álvaro Aranda. 2021. Public service interpreting and translation in Spain. In *Training public service interpreters and translators: A European perspective*, ed. Štefková, Marketa Kerremans, Koen, and Benjamin Bossaert, 71–87.

Leanza, Yvan. 2005. Role of community interpreters in pediatrics as seen by interpreters, physicians and researchers. *Interpreting* 7 (2): 167–192.

Lemus Riscanevo, Paula, Sonia Carreño Moreno and Mauricio Arias Rojas. 2019. Conspiracy of silence in palliative care: a concept analysis. *Indian Journal of Palliative Care* 25(1): 24–29.

Marian, Viorica, and Margarita Kaushanskaya. 2004. Self-construal and emotion in bicultural bilinguals. *Journal of Memory and Language* 51: 190–201.

Mesa, Anne Marie. (2000). The cultural interpreter: an appreciated professional. Results of a study on interpreting services: Client, healthcare worker and interpreter points of view. In *The critical link 2: Interpreters in the community*, ed. Roda Roberts, Silvana E. Carr, Diana Abraham and Aideen Dofour. Amsterdam/Filadelfia: John Benjamins.

Nelson, Bryn. 2018. Left in the dark at the end of life: Miscommunication and a lack of planning can lead to avoidable confusion, stress, and pain for dying patients and their families. *Cancer Cytopathology* 126 (3): 151–152.

Neymeyer, Robert and Melissa Smigelsky. 2018. *Grief therapy. Oxford research encyclopaedia.* USA: Oxford University Press.

Orellana, Marjorie Faulstich, Lisa Dorner and Lucila Pulido. 2003. Accessing assets: Immigrant youth's work as family translators or para-phrasers. *Social Problems* 50: 505–524.

Orellana, Marjorie Faulstich. 2009. *Translating childhoods: Immigrant youth, language, and culture.* New Brunswick, New Jersey: Rutgers University Press.

Pérez Estevan, Elena. 2022. La interpretación sanitaria en final de vida desde la perspectiva de su necesidad ante el impacto de la COVID. In De la hipótesis a la tesis: traductología y lingüística aplicada, ed. Miguel Ibañez Rodríguez, Carmen Cuéllar Lázaro and Paola Masseau, 547–563.

Pöchhacker, Franz. 2001. Quality assessment in conference and community interpreting. *Meta* 46 (2): 410–425.

Pöchhacker, Franz (ed.). 2015. *Routledge encyclopaedia of interpreting studies.* London: New York: Routledge. https://doi.org/10.4324/9781315678467.

Pozo Triviño, María Isabel del. 2017. The right of gender violence victims and survivors to quality translation and interpreting according to legislation. *The SOS-VICS contribution* 23–46.

Roberts, Roda. 1997. Community interpreting today and tomorrow. In 2003 La evaluación de la calidad en interpretación: Investigación, ed. Ángela Collados Aís, Mª Manuela Fernández Sánchez and Daniel Gile, 7–28. Granada: Comares.

Shlesinger, Yael. 2005. Vicarious traumatization among interpreters who work with torture survivors and their therapists. *Chicago School of Professional Psychology* 35: 152–172.

Silva, Milagros, Margaux Genoff, Alexandra Zaballa, Sarah Jewell, Stacy Stabler, Francesca Gany and Lisa Diamond. 2016. Interpreting at the end of life: A systematic review of the impact of interpreters on the delivery of palliative care services to cancer patients with limited English proficiency. *Journal of Pain and Symptom Management* 51(3): 569–580. ISSN 0885-3924. https://doi.org/10.1016/j.jpainsymman.2015.10.011.

Siyu Wu, Margaret and Shail Rawal. 2017. It's the difference between life and death: the views of professional medical interpreters on their role in the delivery of safe care to patients with limited English proficiency. *Plos One* 12: 10. https://doi.org/10.1371/journal.pone.0185659.

Splevins, Katie, Keren Cohen, Stephen Joseph, Craig Murray and Jake Bowley. 2010. Vicarious posttraumatic growth among interpreters. *Qualitative Health Research* 20: 1705–1716.

Teegen, Finn, and C. Goennenwein. 2002. Posttraumatic stress disorder of interpreters for refugees. *Verhaltenstherapie and Verhaltensmedizin* 23: 419–436.

Valero Garcés, Carmen and Elena Alcalde Peñalver. 2021. Empathy in PSI: Where we stand and where to go from here. *Fitispos International Journal* 8(1): 17–27.

Valero Garcés, Carmen. 2021. A place for the human factor in the midst of the COVID-19 pandemic. As a way of introduction. In *The human factor in PSIT*, ed. Carmen Valero Garcés and Elena Alcalde Peñalver, 1–8. Fitispos International Jounal.

Vigor, Jana. 2012. *Vicarious trauma and the professional interpreter. The trauma and mental health report*. American Translators Associations. https://www.atanet.org/interpreting/vicarious-trauma-and-interpreters/.

Wadensjö, Cecilia. 2001. Interpreting in crisis: The interpreters' position in therapeutic encounters. In *Triadic exchanges. Studies in dialogue interpreting*, ed. Ian Mason, 71–85. Manchester: St. Jerome.

Weisskirch, Robert. 2007. Feelings about language brokering and family relations among Mexican American early adolescents. *Journal of Early Adolescence* 27 (4): 545–561.

Elena Pérez Estevan holds a degree in Translation and Interpreting (University of Alicante), a Master's Degree in Intercultural Communication, Public Service Interpreting and Translation (University of Alcalá) and a Master's degree in Medical and Healthcare Translation (Jaume I University, Castellón). She obtained a Ph.D in 2022 in translation studies focusing on end-of-life interpreting. She also completed a course in integrative-relational counselling in grief and loss at IPIR Institute (Barcelona). She is a professor and researcher at the university of Alicante in the Translation and Interpreting department. She has worked as a visiting professor at University of Alcalá. Her research interests include EoL interpreting, psychotherapy, public service interpreting training and quality and communication skills. She has extensive professional experience working as a medical interpreter in different hospitals in Spain for public and private institutions. Member of INCOGNITO research group at University of Alicante. Author of several papers and book chapters in national and international journals.

Analysis of Audio Transcription Tools with Real Corpora: Are They a Valid Tool for Interpreter Training?

Encarnación Postigo Pinazo and Laura Parrilla Gómez

1 State of the Art

This study includes a brief analysis of the impact of new technologies on interpreting practice and the emergence of interpreting tools designed for research and subsequently applied to training. The last part presents a case study sample of the use of speech-to-text technologies to support healthcare interpreters and assesses their quality.

The use of information and communication technologies (ICT) in the field of interpreting has traditionally been researched for simultaneous and conference interpreting, leaving aside its use in public services. However, in the last decade, ICTs have taken on a very important role in healthcare, legal, police and social contexts (Valero Garcés 2018).

The research presented in this study has been (partially) carried out in the framework of the research project "Multi-lingual and Multi-domain Adaptation for the Optimisation of the VIP system" (VIP II, ref. no. PID2020-112818 GB-I00, 2021–2025, Spanish Ministry of Science and Innovation) and within the University Institute for Research in Multilingual Linguistic Technologies (IUITLM-University of Málaga).

The original version of this chapter was revised: The author names and affiliations have been corrected. The correction to this chapter is available
https://doi.org/10.1007/978-981-99-2961-0_10

E. Postigo Pinazo (✉)
University of Málaga, Málaga, Spain
e-mail: epostigo@uma.es

L. Parrilla Gómez
University Pablo de Olavide, Seville, Spain
e-mail: lpargom@upo.es

R. Lázaro Gutiérrez and C. Álvaro Aranda (eds.), *New Trends in Healthcare Interpreting Studies*, New Frontiers in Translation Studies,
https://doi.org/10.1007/978-981-99-2961-0_9

On the one hand, there are the new modalities for the professional practice of interpreting that, together with the new tools and mobile apps facilitate the day-to-day practice of public service interpreting. On the other hand, in the field of research, we highlight the use of corpus analysis and terminology extraction tools that have become a valuable tool for establishing patterns, analysing terminology and recreating situations similar to real life that, in the future, could be used to train future interpreters.

As a prime example let us consider remote interpreting (RI) or also known as teleinterpreting (Parrilla Gómez 2006) or (tele)phone interpreting (Kelly 2008), whose use has increased exponentially with the health situation caused by COVID-19. Public service providers have limited the use of face-to-face care to urgent and necessary cases by resorting to telemedicine and teleconsultations as a priority means of patient care. In this respect, teleinterpretation or telephone interpreting has become the only form of patient-healthcare provider communication in these pandemic years, not only for foreigners but also for speakers of the same language.

This modality, which dates back to the 1970s in Australia and led in its early days to the emergence of companies such as Language Line in the United States (Kelly 2008, p. 5), has been used in a variety of everyday and business contexts, from public services to private companies with a large number of foreign clients. Typically, the public service or company contracts telephone interpreting services with a telephone interpreting provider. The user has a card with a language code to contact the interpreter directly or a device already programmed with each key assigned to a language.

The advantages of working in this way for freelance interpreters are numerous, especially the fact that they can work from home, organising their working hours and being able to combine it with translation work or household chores. However, the interpreter must maintain a series of standards in order to provide quality work, such as, for example, receiving the call in a room isolated from noise, having the telephone nearby so as not to delay the answer to the call, and even so, the lack of availability of the interpreter in risky situations, especially when working with freelance interpreters, can have serious consequences.

In recent years, the use of ICT has gone hand in hand not only with remote interpreting (in which the interpreter may not be physically present in the same space as the user or the provider), but also with the use of devices or materials that help teleinterpreters in their professional life. We are no longer talking about online glossaries, but about mobile applications that, at the click of a button, provide a resource to support the interpreter's work. Universal Doctor Speaker[1], Health Communication[2] or Tradassan[3] have made it easier to search for specialised terms, information on specialties, or even routine questions for certain specific situations such as the triage

[1] https://www.universaldoctor.com/.

[2] https://www.natcom.org/communication-currents/translation-progress-health-communication-app-goes-live.

[3] https://apps.apple.com/es/app/mitradassan/id897901563.

room, replacing the traditional glossaries or information sheets on clinical processes that were used to prepare for interpreting.

These advances have been complemented by Computer-assisted interpreting (CAI), a new model in which software specifically designed to meet the interpreter's needs, especially in terms of terminology and information management, is used (Prandi 2020). These resources that have started to be used mainly for conference interpreting such as InterpretBank,[4] LookUp[5] or Intragloss help prepare specialised assignments, manage terminology and access them in the booth. Thanks to Artificial Intelligence, smart design and cutting-edge technologies have become an aid to the preparation phase by allowing glossaries to be printed or exported. Some of them, such as InterpretBank and Boothmate[6] also allow quick access from the booth (Fantinuoli 2016).

Following Ortiz and Cavallo (2018), the available CAI tools can be categorised into three types: training, preparation and interpreting. There are also tools that have been specifically designed for interpreting. These tools are currently being used not only for the professional practice but also for university programs.

As for the use of speech, some of these tools also integrate automatic speech recognition (ASR) such as InterpretBank. Tools that allow speech recognition or convert speech to text are also very useful when it comes to automatically transcribing speech to text, such as AudioNote, Voice Dictation and Voice Pro.

In this regard, it is necessary to talk about machine interpreting (MI), since in the coming years it will acquire an important role (although probably in the form of simultaneous interpreting) with the development of speech-to-speech systems. In these systems, a device captures human speech in a source language, searches for equivalents against pre-recorded sequences in a target language and reproduces such a sequence (Ortiz and Cavallo 2018, p. 16).

Translation Memories and Computer-Assisted Translation have become the subject of much research. In the context of interpreting, computer-assisted interpreting is a relatively new field (Corpas Pastor 2018), mostly based on theory and little on interpreting practice. Not only is such research scarce, but it is mainly focused on conference interpreting and not on interpreting in public services.

Although research such as Biagini (2015), Prandi (2015), Fantinuoli (2016) have focused on the results of using these tools (interpreter's cognitive process, level of anxiety, concentration), studies focused on speech recognition tools have been devoted mainly to contexts different to the healthcare sector, such as Del Rio et al. (2021) to financial situations. However, it is thanks to the emergence of research projects such as SHIFT,[7] VIP I[8] and VIP II and the compilation of both oral and written corpora with situations recreated in hospital contexts and the search for

[4] https://www.interpretbank.com/site/.

[5] http://www.lookup-web.de/introduction/index.html.

[6] https://apps.apple.com/es/app/boothmate-glossary-lookup/id1114285611.

[7] https://www.shiftinorality.eu/.

[8] http://www.lexytrad.es/vip/site/.

specialised glossaries that interesting tools will be created and become devices adapted to the interpreter in these contexts.

Shift for Orality is an Eramus + project whose aim is set at "developing a comprehensive solution for training in remote interpreting in Higher Education and Lifelong Learning, through the cooperation of a European network of universities offering interpreting programmes and interpreting service providers". As a result of this project, resources, manuals and material for the training of remote interpreters have been compiled.

In this respect, the enormous contribution being made by the LEXYTRAD[9] research group at the University of Málaga, which has been working for several years on different projects covering interpreting in the context of public services, including VIP I, should be highlighted. The main objective was the creation of a working station for interpreters with corpora, glossaries and dictionaries to improve the work of teachers, students and professional interpreters in all phases of the interpreting process (Corpas Pastor 2021). They are currently in the preparation phase of VIP II, with the aim of not only working on tools to help interpreters in the medical context, but also in other contexts such as the legal one.

The SmarTerp Project,[10] funded by the European Union in the framework of EIT Digital BP2021 develops a Remote Interpretation system using Computer Aided Interpretation tools. As a novelty, it is not only intended to become a tool for interpreters alone, but also for conference organisers and language service providers (Fossati 2021, p. 6).

Despite all these advances that are being made at the university level, the tools created or future ones will have to be tested with real speeches in which there are different accents, interruptions, with a high load of specialised terminology and, above all, with the difficulty that comes with interpreting in hospitals in terms of emotions and cultural elements.

2 Methodology

This study will focus on tools for the professional practice of interpreters in public services. The information has been obtained from a corpus of real recordings obtained in a hospital context involving the participation of healthcare staff, doctors, nurses, patient or their relatives and a volunteer interpreter who also usually helps in the institution has been used. The corpus is part of the study by Parrilla Gómez (2014) in which various aspects of the interpreters' production in hospital interactions were analysed.

The reason for choosing this corpus is mainly justified by the fact that it does not deal with recreated or simulated, fictitious situations, but with real conversations that have taken place in public services. This characteristic means that the various factors

[9] http://www.lexytrad.es/es/.

[10] https://smarter-interpreting.eu/theproject/.

that come into play in a conversation, such as noise, interruptions, pauses, etc., make it difficult to analyse for the transcription tools subject of this study.

The participants in the study are people who have already been in situations where they have had to deal with the language barrier and, for the most part, have had to resort to an interpreter. The interpreter, although working on a voluntary basis, is also used for provider-user interactions. For the purpose of naming the participants, the following letters have been assigned to each speaker: interpreter (I), doctor/nurse, public service (PS), patient (P), relative (R).

The contexts chosen are hospital consultations and visits by the doctors to the patients where they are informed about procedures and health conditions. The reason for this choice is based on the occurrence of specialised terminology and the structure of the interview between the two parties, in which questions and answers play a major role.

As for transcription tools, Otter.ai and Amberscript have been used. Previous studies have researched into tools more specifically aimed at interpreters (Gaber and Corpas Pastor 2019) but, unlike the devices and software mentioned at the beginning of the chapter, these are free online tools that are easily accessible to the user and can be an interesting option for the practice of future interpreters. The following table compares some of the advantages and disadvantages of each of them (Table 1).

Finally, for those fragments of conversations where Spanish has been used, a literal translation is provided for better comparison with the translation provided by the tool.

Table 1 Tool comparison

Tool	Advantages	Disadvantages
Otter.ai	Transcription with high % accuracy in small rooms and low noise levels Users can export the transcript and share the text The audio can be played while the transcript text is being checked Different speakers are assigned "Speaker 1," "Speaker 2" etc., and you can add contact names for the "voiceprint" if you know who each speaker is	Free version only 30 min of recording For dialogues with many interruptions, different accents and noise, the work of post-editing is greater
Amber Script	Users can export transcripts in Text, SRT, VTT and many other formats, with optional timestamps and speaker distinction Audio can be connected to the text in our online editor, where you can review, highlight and search with ease	Free version only 10 min of recording It is necessary to choose the language of the recording (difficult for interactions with interpreters where more than one language is spoken)

3 Results

After using the tools to analyse the recordings, the transcriptions and their corresponding translation produced by these websites were analysed and compared with a manual transcription made by the authors. For the purposes of this study, only the fragments considered relevant for the interpreter's work and future training have been selected.

REC01: English < > Spanish.

Context: Neonate.

Speakers: Paediatrician (PS), father (R), interpreter (I).

Tool: Otter ai (Table 2).

The two important pieces of information in this first part, the paediatrician's visit to the father of the two premature babies, have been accurately translated and transcribed, we highlight "no change", "stable", and, although the last sentence is poorly expressed and the programme has not been able to reproduce "weight stagnation", it is possible to extract this information from "didn't come in to come into the weight" (Table 3).

Table 2 Example of transcription with Otter ai

Otter ai	Manual transcription
	(PS) Dile que están **estables**…Que no ha habido ningún cambio *(Tell him they are stable…there has been no change)*
	(PS) Y que bueno están…tienen un poco **de estancamiento ponderado**, de estancamiento de peso *(And…well, they have some weighted stagnation, some weight stagnation)*
And suddenly it was **no change** no change at all so **stable** they didn't come in to come **into the weight**	

Table 3 Example of transcription with Otter ai

Otter ai	Manual transcription
	(PS) Las **constantes son completamente normales**. Que están evolucionando dentro de lo normal para un neonato *(Vitals are completely normal. They are evolving within the normal range for a newborn)*
Everything **is normal and vital signs** as they are pretty mature that's completely normal normal situation feeding valves	

Again, in the doctor's next intervention, "vitals are completely normal" has been captured by the tool (Table 4).

In this English-to-English transcription, we can see that the one provided by Otter ai is almost exact, especially in the important question about his wife's discharge from hospital.

REC02: English < > Spanish.

Context: Discharge report.

Speakers: Doctor (PS), patient (P), interpreter (I).

Tool: Amber script (Table 5).

In this extract the idea of following the "normal" diet that the patient was on before being admitted may still be maintained, and in this respect the tool has been able to convey that information. The same is true for "elastic stocking" which, although the tool has not provided "compression", has used the word "support", so the idea

Table 4 Example of transcription with Otter ai

Otter ai	Manual transcription
	(R) They only thing I want to know is my wife is **being released tomorrow**. How long does he think before they can be…
I know the wall I want to know is wife **to be released tomorrow** How long does it take before they can be	

Table 5 Example of transcription with Amber script

Amber script	Manual transcription
	(PS) Este es el **informe de alta** ¿vale? aquí pone lo que ha tenido en este ingreso las pruebas que se le han hecho… La **dieta habitual** que es la que sigue normalmente ambulación con **media elástica de comprensión fuerte** hasta la rodilla durante dos años y el **sintrom**, que es un **anticoagulante** de 4 miligramos (*This is the discharge report, OK? here you can see what he has had during this admission, the tests that have been done…* *The usual diet, which is the one he normally follows, ambulation with a strong elastic compression stocking up to the knee for two years and sintrom, which is an anticoagulant*)
This is your **medical report** and the tests that you have got to have. Then if your diet is the **normal diet**, whatever your usual diet is, you should walk with your **strong elastic support stocking** now up to the knee. You've got to have **syndrome**, which is an **anticoagulant**	

of using a knee-length stocking for support has been achieved. However, the term “simtrom" was not recognised, although the description provided by the doctor was (Table 6).

In hospital discourse, especially in discharge reports, accurate information about medication, appointments and check-ups and other instructions is essential. This tool has translated and transcribed the information about the patient’s next visit and, in addition, has included the next test the patient has to undergo.

REC03: English < > Spanish.

Context: Doctor’s visit to patient.

Speakers: Doctor (PS), patient (P), interpreter (I).

Tool: Amber script (Table 7).

In the following conversation, in which the doctor wants to clarify with the patient what tests he had previously undergone, the doctor wants to emphasise that he did not undergo an X-ray of the lungs, but a bone scan. The programme transcribes this as “bone density”, and also transmits the clarification as to what kind of test was performed (“not a test for your lungs”) (Table 8).

Although the accuracy of the above extract is not as great as elsewhere, this is an example where “lung” and “inflammable” have been recognised.

REC04: English < > Spanish.

Context: Social Service’s visit to patient.

Speakers: Social Services (PS), patient (P), interpreter (I).

Tool: Otter ai (Table 9).

At the next visit, the social worker tries to explain to the patient what possibilities she has once she leaves the hospital. She wants to offer them the possibility of a person to help them at home, but they will have to pay privately. “You’re paying” and “go home and help” have been captured by the tool.

REC05: English < > Spanish.

Context: Doctor’s visit to patient.

Speakers: Doctor (PS), patient (P), interpreter (I).

Table 6 Example of transcription with Amber script

Amber script	Manual transcription
	(PS) Eh…luego…pedirá cita en consulta externa en **medicina interna en el plazo de seis meses** previamente se le realizará **ecografía doppler** cuya petición se adjunta (*You will then... make an appointment for an outpatient appointment in internal medicine within six months beforehand for a doppler ultrasound scan, the request is enclosed*)
Two appointments. One is to come back and see the doctor, the **internal medicine doctor**, in **six months time**. And before you come to see him an appointment for the **Echo Doppler**, which is here	

Table 7 Example of transcription with Amber script

Amber script	Manual transcription
	(PS)… vamos a ver bien. Tengo un informe de la prueba que se hizo en ______________ y en la que pone que la… porque la prueba que se hizo no es del del **tórax** es de los huesos eh… entonces es una **gammagrafía ósea**. En la gammagrafia ósea, que tampoco se lo hemos pedido nosotros sino el urólogo, es para ver si tenía algún alguna lesión del tumor de la próstata en los huesos y dice que no…que es normal ¿vale? *(… let's have a good look. I have a report of the test that was done at ______________ and in which it says that the… because the test that was done is not of the thorax but of the bones… so it is a bone scan. In the bone scan, which we didn't ask it for either but the urologist did, it was to see if he had any lesion of the prostate tumour in the bones and it said that he didn't…that it was normal, right?)*
OK, all right. She said that the test that you have done in ________ was not a test was not a test for your lungs or anything like that. It is a test for the bone. It was like a bone density. It was a **bone density** to see if current problems were. Your prostate and influenced are going to add anything to it, had had anything to do with your bones and your bones are in perfect condition, OK?	

Table 8 Example of transcription with Amber script

Amber script	Manual transcription
	(PS)… lo que se veía en el **pulmón** era una zona en la que parte de su pulmón se veía **inflamado**
… look at **lung**. You have zone in like a very part, mostly **inflammable**	

Tool: Otter ai (Table 10).

This example of a conversation between doctor and patient was chosen because of the background noise in the room. This corroborates that the Otter ai tool failed to accurately capture some of the key elements of the conversation (bladder, the months).

And just as in quieter conversations the tool was able to pick up the interpreter's and patient's speech in English more accurately, in this case this was not the case due to the noise level in the room.

Table 9 Example of transcription with Otter ai

Amber script	Manual transcription
	(PS)Tenemos otra opción que también sería de ayuda a domicilio una persona que vaya a casa como va esta chica pero sería de forma privada que lo tendréis que pagar vosotros (*We have another option which would also be to have a home person coming to your home as this girl is doing, but it would be a private service that you would have to pay for*)
Most, okay, also have other possibility that is **other person** that would go to home and help **home assistance**. **You're paying the person** price	

Table 10 Example of transcription with Otter ai

Otter ai	Manual transcription
	(PS)…se le puso una nefrostomía percutánea que es un tubito en el riñón el mes pasado y ahora lo que se le ha hecho es una RTU vesical que es una limpieza de la vejiga (*she had a percutaneous nephrostomy which is a small tube in the kidney last month and now she has had a bladder TUR which is a cleansing of the bladder*)
I think that have also questions and syllabus for a **nephrostomy Titania** because a tubit kidney pasado era Oxyelite Vesica Okay…	

REC05: English < > Spanish.
Context: Doctor's visit to patient.
Speakers: Doctor (PS), patient (P), interpreter (I).
Tool: Otter ai (Table 11).

Although the tool captures "a medication to look after", it nevertheless omits key words such as "leg" (lace) and the name of the medication "segurio" (Seguril).

Table 11 Example of transcription with Otter ai

Otter ai	Manual transcription
	(I) … Ok, alright ________ she's going to put in Seguril which is a medication to look after your legs they're very swollen, yeah?
all right choose **segurio** Which is a medication to look after your **lace** three swelling yeah	

The examples mentioned here have been extracted for their relevance to the key ideas and for showing the usefulness of the selected tools. Throughout the analysis of the transcriptions, certain difficulties were observed that prevented the devices from capturing and transcribing part of the conversations with a certain degree of accuracy.

To analyse the difficulties encountered, we will use some categories of the typology established by Fantinuoli (2017, p. 4):

- Use of spoken language: as they are formal encounters but still a dialogue between three people, it is a spontaneous discourse, with hesitations, repetitions, changes of subject in the same conversation, etc. This difficulty was evident when it came to assigning parts of speech to one speaker or another. Parts of speech belonging to different speakers were assigned by the tool to a single speaker.

  REC04: Speaker 1 think you need somebody from noon onwards to help you? I do because I'm 86 I'm not very strong. Okay if I guess he could get a…. (2 speakers take part in this example: Speaker 1 (Interpreter) Speaker 2 (Patient) but the tool assigned this excerpt to just one Speaker.
- Variant of the language used: English, as a lingua franca, is the language used by the interpreter, who in all cases is not a native speaker. The varieties of pronunciation are a challenge for these tools because not all of them are prepared to pick up the different accents of the same language. In our study, the problem came mainly from the different languages that may appear in the discourse, in this case, Spanish and English. While the patient and interpreter's productions have been transcribed with a very high percentage of accuracy, those of the public service provider have shown some incoherence.
- Background noise: as mentioned at the beginning, noise is an important factor in teleinterpretation, but in the face-to-face context it is also for the tools analysed. Although the corpus was collected using a tape recorder at a certain distance from the speakers, as the doctor visited patients or relatives in hospital rooms or consulting rooms, this may have limited the recognition of certain parts of speech.
- Continuous speech: as Fantinouli states (2017, p. 4), ASR faces the challenge of recognition of word boundaries. This has been observed during our research when Spanish was used:

  REC03: Speaker 1*:* (Transcription by Otter ai) Don't rush to the doctor, which he had before said that know nothing on the X-ray, and or don't do this for you anymore. And the figures are always going to say when you come back from international

  Dice que la vez anterior que estuvo aquí el médico le dijo que estaba muy bien que no tenía nada y que no quería volver a verle pero cuando volvió de Inglaterra…

  (He says that the last time he was here the doctor told him that he was fine, that he had nothing and that he didn't want to see him again, but when he returned from England…)

- Ambiguity: In the samples analysed, several examples of this ambiguity and situations where the tools have identified one term for another have been found. For example, *syndrome* instead of *simtrom.*

4 Conclusion

At the end of the study, it became clear that the rise of remote interpreting and computer-assisted interpreting has led to the use of new technologies and has become an additional, even necessary, resource for professional interpreters who work remotely. Until now, this digital assistance has come in the form of mobile applications and online resources, but this study has shown that transcription tools can become another possible avenue for professional interpreters and, in the future, incorporated in university programs.

Previous studies among professional interpreters on the use of remote interpreting, computer-assisted interpreting or automatic interpreting show a variety of opinions. On the one hand, remote interpreting has a higher level of acceptance (SHIFT 2018), probably because it is a widely recognised modality with many years of experience and practice.

On the other hand, while some of these tools may improve the interpreter's work on accuracy issues, the study by Wang and Wang (2019) shows that they may increase the cognitive load of interpreters, especially those with less experience, and may also cause more disadvantages for those with a lower level of linguistic proficiency.

Our study aimed to choose a small representative sample of real recordings to test these devices and check their accuracy and thus their possible use in the field of public service interpreting.

The two tools chosen, Otter ai and Amber script, were chosen because of the simplicity of registration for a normal user, although there are limitations in terms of the number of minutes/recordings allowed for free registration. We are also aware that zero-cost transcription tools could not provide adequate assurances around the confidentiality of the data (Da Silva 2021) but the samples used did not contain any personal data of the participants.

The analysis performed is fast, providing a transcript that can be exported in different formats, not only in .doc or .pdf, but also allows the option of creating subtitles from the analysed recordings. In addition, both also offer the possibility of editing the transcript while listening to the audio, a very interesting option for the process of extracting terminology, syntax and expressions with speeches in the pre-interpretation phase of interpreting.

Amber script allows the option to choose the language of the recording which can be a useful option for analysing linguistic corpora of different languages but similar contexts such as specialty consultations, usual routine procedures such as discharge reports or guided dialogues of consultations to gather patient data.

The results showed that both tools, despite their limitations, captured and transcribed the most relevant information in short recordings with simple sentences and low background noise levels, especially specialised terminology, dates, and procedures. However, limitations have arisen with speeches with background noise, interruptions, and longer sentences.

For these situations, the same tools are offering troubleshooting guides[11] for certain obstacles such as background noise (and its possible solution with third-party noise cancellation software, for example). They also offer the possibility to "train the tool" for slang or proper nouns.

The authors are aware of the limitation of the tools analysed due to the number of minutes of analysis offered in their free version and it is therefore recommended for future research to expand the number of tools as well as the number of real samples analysed. However, all these obstacles could be solved in the future with more efforts aimed at improving these tools and using different corpora from a variety of contexts. The evaluation of these tools could also be improved with the use of World Error Rate (WER) or post-editing (PE) methods (Papadopoulou, et al. 2021, p. 199) and, above all, more research between the Automatic Speech Recognition industry and academia (Szymański et al. 2020).

Although the sample was small, we believe that it is representative of the potential of these tools with real speeches. It is necessary to continue testing audio transcription software and devices in order to turn them into another tool in the interpreter's work, in the same way that text search or terminology management devices are currently used. Having these systems included in university programs for interpreters' training should be a reality since we really need to ensure that graduates are fully prepared for the interpreting market (Donovan 2006, p. 1).

However, research on new technologies needs to be performed "not only on the basis of naturalistic methods (such as corpus analysis), but empirical experiments should be conducted also in stringently controlled experimental conditions" (Fantinuoli 2018, p. 170). Studies such as those by Cariello et al. (2021) where Biomedical Named Entity Recognition tools aim to identify and classify biomedical concepts could become a valuable source to complement studies with corpora obtained in real encounters to train speech recognition tools.

To achieve this goal, it is necessary firstly to highlight the status of public services and the role that computer-assisted interpreting can play in contexts such as hospitals. Secondly, although there are certain actions to give more importance to machine and computer-assisted interpreting such as the Strategic Plan for Interpreting 2020–2024 of the European Commission's General Directorate[12] to achieve a shift of conference interpreting towards cloud-based platforms, speech recognition and automatic transcription tools (Karaban 2021), few efforts are being made in the field of public services. Thanks to projects such as VIP I and VIP II, tools for computer-assisted interpreting will play a more important role in the work of professional interpreters and in the training of future interpreters.

---

[11] https://help.otter.ai/hc/en-us/articles/4403627500951-Troubleshooting-audio-problems.

[12] https://ec.europa.eu/info/system/files/scic_sp_2020-2024_en.pdf.

References

Biagini, G. 2015. Glossario cartaceo e glossario elettronico durante l'interpretazione simultanea: Uno studio comparativo. Master's Dissertation, Università di Trieste.

Carmella Cariello, M., A. Lenci, R. Mitkov. 2021. A comparison named entity recognition models in the biomedical domain. In *TRITON. translation and interpreting technology online*, 76–84. http://triton-conference.org/proceedings/. Accessed 6 Jun 2022.

Corpas Pastor, G. 2018. Tools for interpreters: The challenges that lie ahead. *Current Trends in Translation Teaching and Learning E* 5: 157–182. http://www.cttl.org/uploads/5/2/4/3/5243866/cttl_e_2018_5. Accessed 20 Jan 2022.

Corpas Pastor, G. 2021. Technology solutions for interpreters: The VIP system hermeneus. *Revista De Traducción e Interpretación* 23: 91–123.

Da Silva, J. 2021. Producing 'good enough' automated transcripts securely: Extending Bokhove and Downey (2018) to address security concerns. In *Methodological innovations*. https://journals.sagepub.com/doi/https://doi.org/10.1177/2059799120987766. Accessed 6 Jun 2022.

Del Rio, M., N. Delworth, R. Westerman, M. Huang, N. Bhandari, J. Palakapilly, Q. McNamara, J. Dong, P. Zelasko, M. Jette. 2021. Earnings-21: A practical benchmark for ASR in the Wild, INTERSPEECH 2021. https://arxiv.org/abs/2104.11348. Accessed 28 Jun 2022.

Donovan, C. 2006. Trends—where is interpreting heading and how can training courses keep up. Paper presented at the future of conference interpreting: training, technology and research. London: University of Westminster, 30 June–1 July 2006.

Fantinuoli, C. 2016. InterpretBank. Redefining computer-assisted interpreting tools. In *Proceedings of the translating and the computer 38 conference*, 42–52. London: Editions Tradulex, London.

Fantinuoli, C. 2017. Speech recognition in the interpreter workstation. In *Proceedings of the translating and the computer 39 conference*, 367–377. London: Editions Tradulex.

Fantinuoli, C. 2018. Computer-assisted interpreting: challenges and future perspectives. In *Trends E-Tools and resources for translators and interpreters*, ed. I. Durán, G. Corpas, 153–174. Liden: Koninklijke Brill Nv.

Fossati, G. 2021. SmarTerp: Applying the User-centered design process in a computer-assited interpreting (CAI) tool. Master's Dissertation, Universidad Politécnica de Madrid.

Gaber, M., and G. Corpas Pastor. 2019. Las tecnologías de interpretación a distancia en los servicios públicos: uso e impacto. In *Interpreting in a Changing World: New Scenarios, Technologies, Training Challenges and Vulnerable Groups/La interpretación en un mundo cambiante: nuevos escenarios, tecnologías, retos formativos y grupos vulnerables*, ed. E. Postigo Pinazo, 65–89. Peter Lang: Berlín, Berna, Bruselas, Nueva York, Oxford, Varsovia, Viena.

Karaban, V., and A. Karaban. 2021. Exploring the potential for CAI implementation in interpreter training in Ukraine. In: *International Research-to-Practice Conference for Translators, Young Scholars and Students "Translation Industry: Theory in Action" (TITA 2020)*, ed. T. Andrienko, S. Potapenko, L. Slavova. Kyiv, Ukraine, December 11–12, 2020.

Kelly, N. 2008. Telephone interpreting. A comprehensive guide to the profession. Victoria: Trafford Publishing.

Ortiz, L.E., and P. Cavallo. 2018. Computer-assisted interpreting tools (CAI) and options for automation with automatic speech recognition. *Tradterm* 32: 9–31.

Papadopoulou, M.M., A. Zaretskaya, E. Mitkov. 2021. Benchmarking ASR systems based on post-editing effort and error analysis. In: *Proceedings of the Translation and Interpreting Technology Online Conference*, 199–207. https://aclanthology.org/2021.triton-1.23.pdf. Accessed 20 Jun 2022.

Parrilla Gómez, L. 2006. Teleinterpreting: The future of community interpreting. In: *Proceedings of the Conference Translation Technologies and Culture*, ed. I. Kemble. University of Portsmouth: Portsmouth.

Parrilla Gómez, L. 2014. El reto de una interpretación comunitaria de calidad: buceo en las necesidades formativas y análisis crítico de un corpus de interacción oral en el contexto biosanitario y de servicios sociales español. Phd. Thesis' Dissertation, Universidad de Málaga.

Prandi, B. 2015. The use of CAI tools in interpreters' training: A pilot study. In: *Proceedings of the translating and the computer 37 conference*. Editions Tradulex: Geneva.
Prandi, B. 2020. The use of CAI tools in interpreter training: where are we now and where do we go from here? inTRAlinea. Availabe via http://www.intralinea.org/specials/article/the_use_of_cai_tools_in_interpreter_training. Accessed 28 Jan 22.
Szymański, P., Żelasko, P., Morzy, M., Szymczak, A., Żyła-Hoppe, M., Banaszczak, J., Augustyniak, L., Mizgajski, J., and Carmiel, Y. 2020. WER we are and WER we think we are. https://arxiv.org/abs/2010.03432v1. Accessed 28 Jun 2022.
Valero-Garcés, C. 2018. TISP y tecnología. Retos en la era digital. In *TISP y tecnología. Retos en la era digital*, ed. C. Valero-Garcés. Servicio de Publicaciones de la Universidad de Alcalá: Alcalá de Henares, 01–12.
Wang, X., C. Wang. 2019. Can computer-assisted interpreting tools assist interpreting? Transletters. *International Journal of Translation and Interpreting* 3: 109–139. https://www.uco.es/ucopress/ojs/index.php/tl/article/view/11575/10973. Accessed 23 Jan 22.

Encarnación Postigo Pinazo holds a Ph.D. in English Philology (University of Málaga). She has held various teaching and management positions in state secondary education institutions and since 2000 she has been a lecturer in the Department of Translation and Interpreting at the University of Málaga where she is a Senior Lecturer with tenure. In addition to her training and research duties, she has also been involved in the coordination of teaching staff and is a founding member of the Research Institute of Multilingual Language Technologies at the University of Málaga (IUITLM). She also participates in the international master's degree European Master's in Technology for Translation and Interpreting (EM TTI). Her research interests are focused on lexicography, specialized translation and interpreting and she has published extensively in these fields. She has coordinated European projects and is also a reviewer of different quality publications and an independent assessor in different higher education organizations.

Laura Parrilla Gómez combines her work as a translator and interpreter in the public and private sector with her post as a Headteacher in a language school and her post as Associate Professor at the University Pablo de Olavide. She graduated from the University of Málaga with a BA in Translation and Interpreting and a PGCE in Modern Languages and continued her training with a Master in Medical Translation and Interpreting, obtaining her PhD with a research about community interpreting in the health and social services context. She worked as an interpreter in the UK for five years where she obtained the Diploma in Public Service Interpreting in Health and has published on the subject of Public Service Interpreting in the health field and teleinterpreting. She was part of the organizing committee of the Critical Link conference in Birmingham. She is a member of the research group "Studies and Training of Specialized discourse and new technologies" from the University of Málaga.

Prandi, B. 2015. The use of CAI tools in interpreters' training: A pilot study. In: *Proceedings of the translating and the computer 37 conference*. Editions Tradulex: Geneva.

Prandi, B. 2020. The use of CAI tools in interpreter training: where are we now and where do we go from here? inTRAlinea. Availabe via http://www.intralinea.org/specials/article/the_use_of_cai_tools_in_interpreter_training. Accessed 28 Jan 22.

Szymański, P., Żelasko, P., Morzy, M., Szymczak, A., Żyła-Hoppe, M., Banaszczak, J., Augustyniak, L., Mizgajski, J., and Carmiel, Y. 2020. WER we are and WER we think we are. https://arxiv.org/abs/2010.03432v1. Accessed 28 Jun 2022.

Valero-Garcés, C. 2018. TISP y tecnología. Retos en la era digital. In *TISP y tecnología. Retos en la era digital*, ed. C. Valero-Garcés. Servicio de Publicaciones de la Universidad de Alcalá: Alcalá de Henares, 01–12.

Wang, X., C. Wang. 2019. Can computer-assisted interpreting tools assist interpreting? Transletters. *International Journal of Translation and Interpreting* 3: 109–139. https://www.uco.es/ucopress/ojs/index.php/tl/article/view/11575/10973. Accessed 23 Jan 22.

Encarnación Postigo Pinazo holds a Ph.D. in English Philology (University of Málaga). She has held various teaching and management positions in state secondary education institutions and since 2000 she has been a lecturer in the Department of Translation and Interpreting at the University of Málaga where she is a Senior Lecturer with tenure. In addition to her training and research duties, she has also been involved in the coordination of teaching staff and is a founding member of the Research Institute of Multilingual Language Technologies at the University of Málaga (IUITLM). She also participates in the international master's degree European Master's in Technology for Translation and Interpreting (EM TTI). Her research interests are focused on lexicography, specialized translation and interpreting and she has published extensively in these fields. She has coordinated European projects and is also a reviewer of different quality publications and an independent assessor in different higher education organizations.

Laura Parrilla Gómez combines her work as a translator and interpreter in the public and private sector with her post as a Headteacher in a language school and her post as Associate Professor at the University Pablo de Olavide. She graduated from the University of Málaga with a BA in Translation and Interpreting and a PGCE in Modern Languages and continued her training with a Master in Medical Translation and Interpreting, obtaining her PhD with a research about community interpreting in the health and social services context. She worked as an interpreter in the UK for five years where she obtained the Diploma in Public Service Interpreting in Health and has published on the subject of Public Service Interpreting in the health field and teleinterpreting. She was part of the organizing committee of the Critical Link conference in Birmingham. She is a member of the research group "Studies and Training of Specialized discourse and new technologies" from the University of Málaga.

Correction to: Analysis of Audio Transcription Tools with Real Corpora: Are They a Valid Tool for Interpreter Training?

Encarnación Postigo Pinazo and Laura Parrilla Gómez

Correction to: Chapter "Analysis of Audio Transcription Tools with Real Corpora: Are They a Valid Tool for Interpreter Training?" in: R. Lázaro Gutiérrez and C. Álvaro Aranda (eds.), *New Trends in Healthcare Interpreting Studies*, New Frontiers in Translation Studies, https://doi.org/10.1007/978-981-99-2961-0_9

The original version of the book was inadvertently published with an incorrect author names and affiliations for the authors in Chapter 9 which has now been corrected. The correction chapter and the book have been updated.

The updated version of this chapter can be found at
https://doi.org/10.1007/978-981-99-2961-0_9

R. Lázaro Gutiérrez and C. Álvaro Aranda (eds.), *New Trends in Healthcare Interpreting Studies*, New Frontiers in Translation Studies,
https://doi.org/10.1007/978-981-99-2961-0_10

www.ingramcontent.com/pod-product-compliance
Ingram Content Group UK Ltd.
Pitfield, Milton Keynes, MK11 3LW, UK
UKHW022211051026
15624UKWH00001B/103
* 9 7 8 9 8 1 9 9 2 9 6 0 3 *